Occupational Medicine

Reproductive Hazards

Guest Editors:

Ellen B. Gold, PhD
B. L. Lasley, PhD
Marc B. Schenker, MD, MPH
Institute of Toxicology and Environmental Health
University of California
Davis, California

Volume 9/Number 3   July–September 1994
HANLEY & BELFUS, INC.   Philadelphia

STATE OF THE ART REVIEWS

Publisher: HANLEY & BELFUS, INC.
210 South 13th Street
Philadelphia, PA 19107
(215) 546-4995
Fax (215) 790-9330

OCCUPATIONAL MEDICINE: State of the Art Reviews is included in *Index Medicus, MEDLINE, BioSciences Information Service, Current Contents* and *ISI/BIOMED.*

OCCUPATIONAL MEDICINE: State of the Art Reviews   **(ISSN 0885-114X)**
July–September 1994   **Volume 9, Number 3**   **(ISBN 1-56053-149-5)**

OCCUPATIONAL MEDICINE: State of the Art Reviews is published quarterly by Hanley & Belfus, Inc., 210 South 13th Street, Philadelphia, Pennsylvania 19107. Second-class postage paid at Philadelphia, PA and at additional mailing offices.

POSTMASTER: Send address changes to OCCUPATIONAL MEDICINE: State of the Art Reviews, Hanley & Belfus, Inc., 210 South 13th Street, Philadelphia, PA 19107.

The 1994 subscription price is $82.00 per year U.S., $92.00 outside U.S. (add $40.00 for air mail).

Occupational Medicine: State of the Art Reviews
Vol. 9, No. 3, July–September 1994

REPRODUCTIVE HAZARDS
Ellen B. Gold, PhD, B. L. Lasley, PhD, and
Marc B. Schenker, MD, MPH, Editors

CONTENTS

Preface   ix
Ellen B. Gold, B. L. Lasley, and Marc B. Schenker

Introduction: Rationale for an Update   363
Ellen B. Gold, B. L. Lasley, and Marc B. Schenker

> More than 104,000 chemical and physical agents have been identified in the workplace, but the effects on reproduction of at least 95% of them have not been assessed. Here, the editors of this volume describe changing demographics in the workplace, which underscore the need for evaluating potential hazards to reproduction. They also review findings regarding occupational reproductive hazards to men and women that have been reported over the past decade.

Issues in Regulatory Protection of Reproductive Health in the Workplace   373
Mari S. Golub and Gerald F. Chernoff

> Provisions of federal laws that protect reproductive health in the workplace and information on recent federal actions that seek to enhance such protection are reviewed. California's Birth Defects Prevention Act and its Proposition 65, regulatory programs that specifically address reproductive toxicity, also are described.

Clinical Approach to Male Reproductive Problems   387
James W. Overstreet

> This review of the currently recommended clinical and laboratory approach to the evaluation of male reproductive problems describes history-taking, physical examination, evaluation of semen, evaluation of abnormalities of the endocrine system, and specialized laboratory tests such as bioassays, biochemical tests of sperm function, and tests for antisperm antibodies.

Occupational Hazards to Male Reproduction   405
Steven M. Schrader and M. Helen Kanitz

> Since the field of reproductive toxicology was firmly established a generation ago, various approaches have been used to study toxicologic effects. The authors detail the reproductive effects that have been observed in a number of population-based studies, case-control studies, standardized fertility ratio studies, cohort studies, and clinical studies.

Clinical Approach to Female Reproductive Problems **415**
Anthony P. Cheung

Conditions of infertility addressed here include ovulatory dysfunction, tubal and pelvic factors, uterine and cervical factors, immunologic factors, and unexplained infertility. A discussion of recurrent loss of pregnancy and antenatal diagnosis completes the chapter.

Methods for Evaluating Reproductive Health of Women **423**
B. L. Lasley and Susan E. Shideler

As opposed to the clinical approach taken in the above chapter, the authors here focus on largely subclinical events of importance to reproductive health that may occur without the awareness of the woman or her physician. Urinary assays that can detect early fetal loss, monitor ovarian function, and monitor pituitary function are described in detail.

Occupational Hazards to Fertility and Pregnancy Outcome **435**
Ellen B. Gold and Elizabeth Tomich

Many diverse substances and other factors encountered in the workplace that have been associated with infertility and spontaneous abortion are addressed in this chapter, including toluene, mercury, organic solvents, noise, shift work, irregular work schedules, stress, dry cleaning chemicals, antibiotics, and many others. Extensive tables detail the results of numerous studies that have assessed the reproductive effects of occupational exposures.

Congenital Malformations Related to Occupational Reproductive Hazards **471**
Lowell E. Sever

Occupational and environmental agents are the suspected cause of at least some of the approximately 60% of birth defects whose etiology is unknown. The author discusses studies of birth defects published since 1988. Studies that examine associations between congenital malformations and both maternal and paternal exposures are included.

Childhood Cancers Associated with Parental Occupational Exposures ... **495**
Ellen B. Gold and Lowell E. Sever

Statistics suggest that environmental and occupational exposures may be at least partially responsible for an increased incidence of cancer in children. The authors describe the latest findings in this area of research and look at the methodologic concerns that arise and how they affect the derivation of causal inferences from such studies.

Workplace Policy on Hazards to Reproductive Health **541**
Cathy L. Saiki, Ellen B. Gold, and Marc B. Schenker

This chapter on workplace policy pays particular attention to the paradox that the worker's right to be free of discrimination in the workplace may conflict with the right to be free of hazards to reproduction. Legal and ethical concerns are discussed, as are issues such as employee counseling, job transfers and reassignments, and screening, monitoring, and surveillance.

Index **551**

CONTRIBUTORS

Gerald F. Chernoff, PhD
Office of Environmental Health Hazard Assessment, Reproductive and Cancer Hazard Assessment Section, California Environmental Protection Agency, Sacramento, California

Anthony P. Cheung, MB BS, MPH, FRACOG, FRCS(C)
Assistant Professor, Department of Obstetrics and Gynaecology, University of Alberta, Edmonton, Alberta, Canada

Ellen B. Gold, PhD
Associate Professor, Division of Occupational/Environmental Medicine and Epidemiology, Department of Internal Medicine, School of Medicine; Institute of Toxicology and Environmental Health, University of California, Davis, California

Mari S. Golub, PhD
Office of Environmental Health Hazard Assessment, Reproductive and Cancer Hazard Assessment Section, California Environmental Protection Agency, Sacramento, California

Mary Helen Kanitz, PhD
Research Biologist, Experimental Toxicology Branch, National Institute for Occupational Safety and Health, Robert A. Taft Laboratories, Cincinnati, Ohio

B. L. Lasley, PhD
Department of Population, Health, and Reproduction, School of Veterinary Medicine; Division of Reproductive Biology, School of Medicine; Institute of Toxicology and Environmental Health, University of California, Davis, California

James W. Overstreet, MD, PhD
Professor, Division of Reproductive Biology, Department of Obstetrics and Gynecology, School of Medicine; Director, Institute of Toxicology and Environmental Health, University of California, Davis, California

Cathy L. Saiki, MS
Division of Occupational/Environmental Medicine and Epidemiology, School of Medicine; Institute of Toxicology and Environmental Health, University of California, Davis, California

Marc B. Schenker, MD, MPH
Professor and Division Chief, Division of Occupational/Environmental Medicine and Epidemiology, Department of Internal Medicine, School of Medicine; Institute of Toxicology and Environmental Health, University of California, Davis, California

Steven M. Schrader, PhD
Chief, Functional Toxicology Section, National Institute for Occupational Safety and Health, Robert A. Taft Laboratories, Cincinnati, Ohio

Lowell E. Sever, PhD
Staff Scientist, Health Risk Assessment Department, Battelle Pacific Northwest Laboratories, Richland, Washington

Susan Elizabeth Shideler, PhD
Associate Research Endocrinologist, Department of Population, Health, and Reproduction, School of Veterinary Medicine; Institute of Toxicology and Environmental Health, University of California, Davis, California

Elizabeth Tomich, BS
Division of Occupational/Environmental Medicine and Epidemiology, School of Medicine; Institute of Toxicology and Environmental Health, University of California, Davis, California

PUBLISHED ISSUES
(available from the publisher)

Vol 2/No 2
Apr.–June 1987

Occupational Pulmonary Disease
Edited by Linda Rosenstock, MD, MPH

Vol 2/No 4
Oct.–Dec. 1987

Workers with Multiple Chemical Sensitivities
Edited by Mark R. Cullen, MD

Vol 3/No 2
Apr.–June 1988

Worker Fitness and Risk Evaluations
Edited by Jay S. Himmelstein, MD, MPH
and Glenn S. Pransky, MD, MPH

Vol 3/No 3
July–Sept. 1988

The Petroleum Industry
Edited by Neill K. Weaver, MD

Vol 3/No 4
Oct.–Dec. 1988

Psychiatric Injury in the Workplace
Edited by Robert C. Larsen, MD, and Jean S. Felton, MD

Vol 4/No 1
Jan.–Mar. 1989

The Management Perspective
Edited by L. Fleming Fallon, Jr., MD, MPH, MBA,
O.B. Dickerson, MD, MPH,
and Paul W. Brandt-Rauf, ScD, MD, DrPH

Vol 4/No 2
Apr.–June 1989

Alcoholism and Chemical Dependency
Edited by Curtis Wright, MD, MPH

Vol 4/No 4
Oct.–Dec. 1989

Problem Buildings
Edited by James E. Cone, MD, MPH
University of California, San Francisco, California
and Michael Hodgson, MD, MPH

Vol 5/No 1
Jan.–Mar. 1990

Hazardous Waste Workers
Edited by Michael Gochfeld, MD, PhD
and Elissa Ann Favata, MD

Vol 5/No 2
Apr.–June 1990

Shiftwork
Edited by Allene J. Scott, MD, MPH

Vol 5/No 3
July–Sept. 1990

Medical Surveillance in the Workplace
Edited by David Rempel, MD, MPH

Vol 5/No 4
Oct.–Dec. 1990

Worksite Health Promotion
Edited by Michael E. Scofield, PhD

Vol 6/No 1
Jan.–Mar. 1991

Prevention of Pulmonary Disease in the Workplace
Edited by Philip Harber, MD, MPH
and John R. Balmes, MD

Vol 6/No 2
Apr.–June 1991

The Biotechnology Industry
Edited by Alan M. Ducatman, MD
and Daniel F. Liberman, PhD

Vol 6/No 3
July–Sept. 1991

Health Hazards of Farming
Edited by D. H. Cordes, MD, MPH
and Dorothy Foster Rea, MS

Vol 6/No 4
Oct.–Dec. 1991

The Nuclear Energy Industry
Edited by Gregg S. Wilkinson, PhD

1994 ISSUES

Occupational Skin Disease
Edited by James R. Nethercott, MD
University of Maryland
Baltimore, Maryland

Occupational Safety and Health Training
Edited by Michael J. Colligan, PhD
National Institute for Occupational
  Safety and Health
Cincinnati, Ohio

Reproductive Hazards
Edited by Ellen B. Gold, PhD,
B. L. Lasley, PhD, and
Marc B. Schenker, MD, MPH

Tuberculosis in the Workplace
Edited by Steven Markowitz, MD
New York University School of Medicine
New York, New York

1993 ISSUES

The Mining Industry
Edited by Daniel E. Banks, MD
West Virginia University
Morgantown, West Virginia

De Novo Toxicants
Edited by Dennis J. Shusterman, MD, MPH
California EPA, Berkeley, California
and Jack E. Peterson, PhD, CIH
Alpine, California

Spirometry
Edited by Ellen A. Eisen, ScD
University of Massachusetts
Lowell, Massachusetts

Women Workers
Edited Dana M. Headapohl, MD
St. Patrick's Hospital
Missoula, Montana

1992 ISSUES

Back School Programs
Edited by Lynne A. White
Director, Practice Management Resources
San Francisco, California

Occupational Lung Disease
Edited by William S. Beckett, MD
Yale University School of Medicine
New Haven, Connecticut
and Rebecca Bascom, MD
University of Maryland School of Medicine
Baltimore, Maryland

Unusual Occupational Disease
Edited by Dennis J. Shusterman, MD, MPH
Berkeley, California
and Paul D. Blanc, MD, MSPH
University of California, San Francisco
San Francisco, California

Ergonomics
Edited by J. Steven Moore, MD
Medical College of Wisconsin
and Arun Garg, PhD
University of Wisconsin–Milwaukee
Milwaukee, Wisconsin

Ordering Information:
Subscriptions for full year and single issues are available from the publisher—
Hanley & Belfus, Inc., 210 South 13th Street, Philadelphia, PA 19107.
Telephone (215) 546-7293; (800) 962-1892. Fax (215) 790-9330.

PREFACE

Over the last few decades, and particularly in the last decade, a number of marked sociological, demographic, and technological changes have occurred in the United States that have had important implications for assessing potential reproductive hazards in the workplace. Most notably these changes include, first, the rapid pace with which increasing numbers of chemicals have been introduced into the workplace and about which relatively little is known of toxicity, particularly reproductive toxicity. Second, the number of women in the work force has increased dramatically, so that the majority of women who are of the ages at which pregnancy is possible are likely to be working. Third, many of these women have entered occupations traditionally held by men, including factory jobs, repair jobs, and service sector positions, which may involve potential exposures to reproductive hazards. However, many of these positions now held by women are often lower-paying, resulting in less access to health care and health education and often providing minimal or no insurance benefits. In addition, with the introduction and widespread use of computer technology and the increasing speed with which computer-aided tasks can be performed, even jobs traditionally held by women, such as secretarial and data entry positions, have become subject to increased stresses associated with pressure for increased productivity in the workplace. Therefore, the role of occupational stress as a potential reproductive hazard is becoming an increasing concern. Fourth, in the clinic and the laboratory, the technology for assessing, diagnosing, and treating reproductive disorders has also improved in recent decades. This has enabled scientific investigators and clinicians to detect adverse reproductive effects of workplace exposures earlier and more completely and accurately. Thus, researchers can now more readily study abnormalities in male and female fertility as well as early pregnancy loss with more sensitive and specific investigative instruments.

The chapters that follow provide detailed reviews of the progress that has been made clinically in assessment, diagnosis, and treatment of male and female reproductive disorders as well as the technological advances that have occurred in the laboratory. Further, a number of the chapters review the occupational reproductive toxicants for men and women that have been identified and studied in recent years and the risks that they pose in the workplace to male and female fertility, to pregnancy, and to risk of childhood cancer, which may well be thought of as an adverse reproductive outcome. In addition, two chapters review the regulatory and workplace policy implications of identifying occupational reproductive toxicants.

The male and female reproductive systems may be uniquely sensitive to the adverse effects of occupational exposures because reproduction is not essential for survival of the organism. Thus, the reproductive systems may be compromised at lower exposure levels than other physiologic systems and may therefore be very sensitive indicators of occupational exposures and hazards. Until recently, however, much of reproductive function, such as gametogenesis, ovulation, gamete transport, fertilization, implantation, and very early pregnancy loss, has been hidden or relatively inaccessible to accurate scientific investigation. With the recent technological advances in the laboratory, many of these previously hidden functions can now be more readily and accurately examined, and with the recent work force changes that have occurred, the identification of occupational reproductive hazards has become increasingly important. This volume provides an up-to-date review of the current state of knowledge in these vital areas.

ELLEN B. GOLD, PhD
B. L. LASLEY, PhD
MARC B. SCHENKER, MD, MPH
Guest Editors

ELLEN B. GOLD, PhD
B. L. LASLEY, PhD
MARC B. SCHENKER, MD, MPH

INTRODUCTION: RATIONALE FOR AN UPDATE

From the Division of Occupational/
Environmental Medicine and
Epidemiology
School of Medicine
and Institute of Toxicology and
Environmental Health (EBG,
MBS)
and
Division of Reproductive
Biology
School of Medicine
and Institute of Toxicology and
Environmental Health (BLL)
University of California
Davis, California

Reprint requests to:
Ellen B. Gold, PhD
Associate Professor
Division of Occupational/
Environmental Medicine and
Epidemiology
Institute of Toxicology and
Environmental Health
University of California
Davis, CA 95616-8648

Supported by a Research Career
Development Award from the Na-
tional Institute of Environmental
Health Sciences (5 K04 ES00202-4)
(EBG).

INCREASING PUBLIC CONCERN REGARDING OCCUPATIONAL AND ENVIRONMENTAL EFFECTS ON REPRODUCTION

At the time of the last review of occupational reproductive hazards in this publication in
1986, a number of occupational and environmental agents had been associated with reduced
fertility.[1] Estimates show that up to 20 million of
workers in the United States are exposed to
toxic materials (not necessarily reproductive
toxicants).[13] Yet the effects on reproduction of at
least 95% of the more than 104,000 chemical
and physical agents in the workplace listed by
the National Institute for Occupational Safety
and Health Registry of Toxic Effects of Chemical
Substances have not been assessed,[5] partly because their rate of introduction into industry far
outpaces the ability of scientists to perform such
evaluations. More than 400 chemicals with
known reproductive effects are covered by federal
occupational health standards,[46] but regulatory
standards are often based on acute health effects
or cancer risk[70] and rarely on reproductive
effects.[19] However, the reproductive system, being
largely nonessential to survival, may be even
more sensitive to the adverse effects of low-level
exposures.[18,30] Further, the physiologic changes
in the respiratory, cardiovascular, and genitourinary tracts during pregnancy may enhance sensitivity to toxic substances.[28]

A further consideration is that while some
toxicants may be banned or have strict limits on

exposures in the United States due to their toxic effects, they may still be manufactured here and exported for use in other countries (e.g., DDT and Mirex) where the exposures may be higher and less regulated.[70] Furthermore, in U.S. regulatory agencies, data on reproductive hazards are often ignored in decision-making.[70]

Meanwhile, of the 3.8 million live births that occur each year in the United States, approximately 274,000 of the babies are of low birthweight (less than 2,500 g, a major risk factor for infant mortality), 375,000 are preterm (fewer than 37 weeks gestation), and 250,000 are born with birth defects, about half of which are considered major and for at least 60% of which the etiology is unknown.[44,70] In addition, 600,000 pregnancies result in miscarriage or fetal death, outcomes that have been associated with occupational exposures but for which the etiology of many is unknown. Further, sperm counts have decreased 30–40% in the past 30 years, the reasons for which are also largely unknown.[63,70] In 1987, the estimated cost of treating infertility in the U.S. was $1 billion, and for treating neurologic and communicative developmental disorders alone, it was $114 billion.[26] While women have unique potential for experiencing adverse reproductive effects from toxic occupational exposures during pregnancy—because they are the ones that have the pregnancies—preconceptional exposures may have toxic effects on both male and female reproduction. Further, identifying occupational effects on reproduction is of fundamental importance because the effects are largely preventable.

Demographic features of the work force have changed in the last four decades and also underscore the importance of evaluating potential occupational hazards to reproduction. In 1989, approximately 119.5 million adults older than 16 were employed in the labor force. About 55 million (46%) of the workers were women, about 39 million of whom ranged in age from 16–44,[41] ages at which they might be considering or undertaking reproduction. This meant that 73% of non-institutionalized civilian women in this age group in 1990 were participating in the labor force, as compared to 88% of men in this age group;[41] the percentage among women was up from 29% in 1950[42] and 66% in 1986.[43] About 80% of men and 84% of women in the labor force were employed in health, technical, service, precision production, operator, or farming occupations—occupations in which they were likely to encounter potentially hazardous exposures.[41] In addition, the median weekly earnings for 16- to 44-year-olds employed full-time in 1989 was $459 for men and $342 for women,[41] and only 16% of the women and 24% of the men belonged to unions.[7] Thus, women in age groups in which conception could occur were more likely than men to be employed in potentially hazardous occupations and in lower paying jobs, which often lead to greater exposure and provide less insurance and access to health care, including gynecologic and prenatal care.[43,59] Furthermore, even jobs traditionally held by women entail significant chemical or physical reproductive hazards,[42] but they tend to be minimally regulated by the Occupational Safety and Health Administration.[34] Also, the proportion of women who work during their first pregnancy has increased over time from 50% in 1966–70 to 65% in 1981–85.[43]

From 1970 to 1990, the number of families maintained by women increased steadily, from 12% to 18%.[17] Thus, a related issue is that of the working poor. From 1987 to 1990, when the official poverty level was an annual income of $13,359 for a family of four, 6.2–6.6 million workers, or 5% of the labor force, (5% of whites, 13% of Hispanics, 12% of blacks, 5% of men, and 6% of women in the labor force) lived in families whose incomes fell below the poverty level.[17] This included 3.4 million full-time workers. The group with the highest percentage of workers living in poverty was single women who maintained families: 17% in 1990 compared with 9% of single men who maintained families, 4% of married men, and 2.4% of married women with families. The majority of the working poor (1.9 of the 3.5 million workers) were married to another worker; the rate of poverty in this group declined from 1970 to 1992.[17] An increased rate of poverty was observed based on the size of the family—from 2% in couples with no children to 29% with five or more children in 1990, and from 5% to 76%, respectively, in families financially supported by women.

MECHANISMS OF REPRODUCTIVE TOXICOLOGY

Reproductive processes are complex; a number of hormones in men and women regulate gametogenesis, fertilization, implantation, embryogenesis, and fetal growth and development.[19] Dysfunction can occur in any phase of the reproductive process and result in any number of disturbances, including male impotence, reductions in number of sperm, reductions in sperm motility and morphology, disturbances in menstrual cycles (reflecting disturbances in ovulatory function[24] and associated with subfertility), miscarriage, preterm birth, low birthweight, or complications of pregnancy. In addition, male-mediated toxicity may occur indirectly by transmission of agents to the mother via seminal fluid or by maternal exposure to agents brought home by the father.[50] Reproductive toxicants may influence these adverse outcomes by interfering with vital cellular structures or functions, such as DNA and protein enzymes, and/or by disrupting necessary endocrine function,[37] as in the inhibition of gonadotropin secretion by DDT and its metabolites[32] or action as estrogen agonists or antagonists by organochlorines,[2] polychlorinated biphenyls,[8] polybrominated biphenyls[55] or kepone.[15] Further, toxic effects are generally accepted to be cumulative in women because they are born with all the ova they will ever have. Although it is generally thought that many toxic reproductive effects in men are transitory due to the relatively rapid turnover and continuous production of sperm, point mutations to male stem cells can cause permanent damage and, thus, effects may accumulate in men as well.[26] Further, some spermatotoxins such as dibromochloropropane (DBCP) may permanently impair spermatogenesis.[10]

IMPROVED KNOWLEDGE OF REPRODUCTIVE BIOLOGY AND TECHNOLOGY

The understanding of basic reproductive biology, methods for assessing reproductive health, and the technologies to overcome infertility have undergone major changes and improvement since the last review on reproductive health in this series was published in 1986. However, despite this progress in technology and reproductive biology, reproductive health is still a major public concern. Infertility among young couples has been increasing, with more than 2 million couples now estimated to be involuntarily childless.[70] Not only does the United States still have one of the highest infant mortality rates among developed countries, sperm counts of American men are decreasing,[63,70] and approximately 10–15% of all pregnancies result in spontaneous abortion prior to the 20th week of gestation.[76] More than 200,000 birth defects are recorded annually in the United States, and about 3% of all infants have major defects, 5% of which have been attributed to a mutant gene.[70] These statistics were enough to prompt the Senate Committee on Governmental Affairs to commission the General Accounting Office to identify possible environmental factors that might be implicated in reduced fertility and birth defects, the extent that putative reproductive toxicants are regulated, the degree that regulations were based on reproductive toxicity, and to determine if current policies are adequate to protect the public from adverse reproductive exposures.[70]

The GAO's study revealed that no federal agency had listed environmental agents suspected to be toxic to human reproduction or development and responded by listing the 30 chemicals that the GAO considered to be of highest concern. Two thirds of the regulations governing these 30 compounds were not based on reproductive toxicity data, but were coincidental to decisions safeguarding the public against cancer and other concerns. The report concluded that the protection currently afforded to the public against reproductive and developmental toxicity is uncertain at best and that protective regulation for the 30 putative reproductive toxins may be insufficient.[70]

This volume includes discussion of reproductive effects of occupational exposures in both men and women. Historically, special consideration has not been given to the effects of occupational exposures on female reproductive health, but it should be and is increasingly now because of recent changes in economics, lifestyle, and demographics. Over the past two to three decades, the role of women's occupational exposures has taken on increasing importance because more women work outside the home than ever before, and many work in industrial settings in which the appearance of new chemicals outpaces the ability to screen them for potential toxicity. Even in nonindustrial settings, the opportunity for women to be exposed to occupational hazards involving ergonomic and other physical stressors has grown proportionally with the use of electronic devices and chemicals in the office. Female reproductive events are dynamic and are often concealed, and we now recognize that very early pregnancies are lost without being detected by either the mother or her physician[76] and that environmental exposures may increase the frequency of such events. New methodologies have been developed to meet these new concerns, and our understanding of female reproduction and the effects of the environment on it is rapidly changing.

The advances in assisted reproductive health technologies have extended the years of potential childbearing of women. The natural fertile life span of women, which was considered to be limited to the third and fourth decades of life, has been extended through exogenous hormone therapy and embryo transfer to postmenopausal women. It is now possible for women to have embryos frozen for later use, and this innovation forces a new definition of the reproductive years of life.

Computerization of semen evaluations has increased the ability to detect abnormalities in male reproduction and has broadened the concepts of male infertility and the effects of male reproductive toxic exposures. Information is now available to suggest that male exposures can both decrease fertility as well as increase the risk of developmental defects.

The greatest progress in reproductive biology over the past 15 years has been in the technologies developed to study female physiology and toxicology. In vitro fertilization, embryo transfer, and artificial insemination have led to a much greater understanding of ovulation, fertilization, and implantation and have provided the basis for techniques that can be extended to field studies. The application of urinary monitoring to assess early pregnancy failure and ovarian function has led to the recognition that preconceptive events relating to menstrual function may be as important as early pregnancy failures in epidemiologic studies of occupational reproductive hazards.

DOCUMENTED EXPOSURES

Exposures in Men

The evidence for a dramatic decrease in semen quality over the comparatively short period of the past 50 years[6] has suggested that environmental and occupational factors may be major contributing causes of the decline and of an associated decrease in fertility.[14] Suggested factors supporting an environmental etiology for the decline include man as the terminal link in the nutrition chain, the acceptance and ubiquitousness of environmental pollution in industrialized countries, and sensitivity of the germinal epithelium to toxic exposures.[14]

Data on toxic exposures to male reproduction continue to be sparse and limited. Most population-based studies lack useful exposure data, and there have been relatively few targeted studies of specific agents. The difficulties in conducting field studies of male reproduction partly explain this situation.[61] Despite these difficulties, there have been several important studies on occupational hazards to male reproduction since the last *State of the Art Reviews* on this subject. The major categories of documented toxic exposure or adverse effects include the heavy metals, solvents, pesticides, and other agricultural chemicals and miscellaneous exposures, such as heat and welding.

One of the first documented male reproductive toxicants, lead, continues to be associated with adverse reproductive effects. Elevated paternal lead exposure, documented by blood levels, was associated with an increased risk of spontaneous abortion in a Finnish case-control study,[35] and another Finnish study provided limited support for an association of occupational exposure to lead in the father and congenital malformations in the offspring.[57] Concern exists about the possible effects on reproduction of exposure to other heavy metals, such as mercury, cadmium, and arsenic; in vitro studies have demonstrated reduced sperm motility from heavy metal exposure.[11] Many industrial environments raise concern about complex exposures, including heavy metals. For example, smelting, chemical factories, and welding may include heavy metal exposures.

The dramatic demonstration in 1977 of infertility among men exposed to dibromochloropropane (DBCP)[75] appropriately focused attention on the effects of pesticides and other agricultural chemicals on male reproduction. A follow-up of DBCP-exposed workers demonstrated that this chemical induced infertility and resulted in permanent azoospermia among affected men.[10] Studies also have demonstrated chlorinated hydrocarbons in seminal fluid and an associated reduction in sperm motility. Studies of Vietnam veterans have suggested that impairment in semen quality may have resulted from exposure to herbicides.[9] Other agricultural chemicals, including ethylene dibromide and carbaryl (Sevin), also have been associated with impaired semen function or male fertility.

Early toxicologic studies demonstrated reproductive toxicity of the ethylene glycol ethers, particularly 2-methoxyethanol, 2-ethoxyethanol, and their acetates.[23,45] More recently, the reproductive toxicity of these agents has been shown in men and women. A case-control study of patients at a fertility clinic found a highly significant association of reduced sperm concentration and other clinical parameters of reduced sperm function with urinary metabolites of ethoxyacetic acid.[71] Other recent studies have also demonstrated an effect of ethylene glycol ethers on semen quality.[52,72] Studies of the adverse reproductive effects associated with male exposure to other glycol ethers and to other organic solvents have been fewer in number but deserve attention because of the common use of these agents in industry.

Other occupational exposures associated with adverse male reproductive effects may involve complex exposures that are not yet understood. For example, a series of recent studies have demonstrated impairment in semen quality and reduced fertility among welders, an occupation associated with potential exposure to excess heat, solvents, heavy metals, and noise.[3,4] The role of stress in this and other occupational exposures also deserves further investigation.

Exposures in Women

Although studies in both sexes are lacking, studies of the occupational reproductive hazards to women have probably been more numerous than those in men because, despite the fact that many reproductive endpoints in women are not readily observable and routinely recorded in occupational medical records (subfertility, delayed conception, early pregnancy loss, menstrual cycle dysfunction), a number of outcomes are fairly readily observable (low birthweight, clinically observed spontaneous abortion, preterm labor) and medically recorded. In addition, techniques for observing reproductive outcomes in women are less invasive than those in men, particularly with recent developments in urinary monitoring for ovarian function and early pregnancy loss. Thus, many studies involving different designs and examining a variety of occupational exposures and potential hazards to women's reproductive function have been conducted since the last issue of *State of the Art Reviews* that examined this topic.

Although studies of some exposures and outcomes (risk of spontaneous abortion, low birthweight or preterm birth with exposure to video display terminals or electromagnetic fields) have shown inconsistent results,[12,20,27,33,40,48,51,54,62,73,74,78] a number of results have been fairly consistent and are quite suggestive of causal relationships. Occupational exposure to solvents appears to increase the risk of dysmenorrhea[47,79] and spontaneous abortions, particularly with exposure to organic solvents.[28,34,67,69,77] Increased risk of adverse reproductive outcomes has also been observed among women who work in agricultural settings but has not been linked to specific exposures.[21,39,53] In addition, physical stressors such as shift work, long hours standing, and lifting have been associated fairly consistently with increased risk of spontaneous abortion or preterm birth.[16,36,38,49] Finally, while complete agreement among studies is lacking, many authors have observed increased risk of subfertility or spontaneous abortion associated with work in medical occupations and with some specific medical exposures, such as nitrous oxide, anesthetic gases, and antineoplastic drugs.[29,38,39,56,58,60,65]

Much remains to be explored in this area of investigation, particularly in efforts to clarify relationships for exposures and outcomes that have shown inconsistent results in the past. These require specific efforts to validate exposures and outcomes with reliable and unbiased measurements, to investigate and control for confounding variables with greater rigor, to consider the effects of multiple comparisons, and to study populations of adequate size to provide for meaningful statistical analyses that can examine potential dose response and timing of exposure effects.

POLICY IMPLICATIONS OF OCCUPATIONAL REPRODUCTIVE HAZARDS

As discussed by Sciarra,[64] to attain reproductive health, the status of women in society must be elevated. As Giacoia[19] states, social and corporate policies regarding reproductive hazards need to focus on removing hazards rather than removing workers, in compliance with Title VII of the Civil Rights Act of 1964 and its amendment, the federal Pregnancy Discrimination Act of 1978. In the Nordic countries, a cooperative project has developed criteria for classifying an agent as a reproductive toxicant if it causes damage to the genotype of the individual, disturbs hormonal regulation of reproductive functions, causes damage in the reproductive organs leading to decreased fertility, disturbs pregnancy or development or health (including childhood cancer) of the offspring, or adversely affects lactation.[68] An agent can be so designated based on epidemiologic studies in which chance and bias were reasonably excluded or, if they were not, it has been shown in at least one species of experimental animals or in supporting toxicologic evidence. While the use of these criteria remain to be established, Finland, Denmark, and Quebec, Canada, have integrated prevention of reproductive hazards into their laws, and the European Community is also undertaking classification of chemical for reproductive toxicity, including adverse effects on sexual behavior, male and female fertility, teratogenicity, and functional and behavioral development of the offspring.[66] In California, Proposition 65 (California Safe Drinking Water and Toxic Enforcement Act) which was passed in 1986, prohibits discharge into drinking water and requires that warnings be provided to persons exposed in the workplace, the environment, or in consumer products to agents that are known to cause cancer or reproductive/developmental toxicity.[25]

CONCLUSION

This volume provides an update of examinations of reproductive hazards reported in the last decade rather than a comprehensive, long-term review. Cautionary discussions regarding methodologic considerations in reviewing such material are also provided, as are reviews of new technologies for measuring reproductive endpoints. This information should also be interpreted against the backdrop of the changing demographics of the U.S. work force and the changing economic and occupational roles of women and of the working poor in this country. The magnitude of chemical and physical agents introduced into the workplace without sufficient knowledge about their reproductive toxicity as well as the burden of adverse reproductive effects and their attendant costs warrant increased regulatory awareness and action, and the large proportion of adverse reproductive effects whose etiology is unknown warrants increased scientific investigation. Technologies that have become available in recent years for measuring reproductive endpoints have improved the ability of researchers to study these outcomes in working populations of men and women. The occupational and health policy and confidentiality and ethical implications of such scientific inquiry also are considered in this volume.

REFERENCES

1. Baird DD, Wilcox A: Effects of occupational exposures on the fertility of couples. Occup Med State Art Rev 1:361–374, 1986.
2. Bitman J, Cecil HC: Estrogenic activity on DDT analogs and polychlorinated biphenyls. J Agr Food Chem 18:1108–1112, 1970.
3. Bonde JP: Semen quality in welders before and after three weeks of non-exposure. Br J Ind Med 47:515–518, 1990.
4. Bonde JP, Hansen KS, Levine RJ: Fertility among Danish male welders. Scand J Work Environ Health 16:315–322, 1990.
5. California Policy Seminar: Reproductive Health Hazards in the Workplace: Policy Options for California. University of California, Berkeley, 1992.

6. Carlsen E, Giwercman A, Keiding N, Skakkebaek NE: Evidence for decreasing quality of semen during the past 50 years. BMJ 305:609–613, 1992.
7. Chavkin W: Closed office building syndrome. In Chavkin W (ed): Double Exposure: Women's Health Hazards on the Job and at Home. New York, Monthly Review, 1984, pp 81–85.
8. Derr SK, Decker J: Alterations of androgenicity in rats exposed to PCBs (Aroclor 1254). Bull Environ Contam Toxicol 21:43–45, 1979.
9. DeStefano F, Annest JL, Kresnow MJ, et al: Semen characteristics of Vietnam veterans. Reprod Toxicol 3:165–173, 1989.
10. Eaton M, Schenker MB, Whorton M, et al: Seven-year follow-up of workers exposed to 1,2-dibromo-3-chloropropane. J Occup Med 28:1145–1150, 1986.
11. Eggert-Kruse W, Rohr G, Jochum R, et al: The effect of heavy metals on the in vitro interaction between human sperm and cervical mucus. Deutsche Medizinische Wochenschrift 117:1383–1389, 1992.
12. Ericson A, Kallen B: An epidemiological study of work with video screens and pregnancy outcome: I. A registry study. Am J Ind Med 9:447–457, 1986.
13. Equal Employment Opportunity Commission, OFCCP: Interpretive guidelines on employment discrimination and reproductive hazards. Federal Register 45:7514–7517, February 1, 1980.
14. Feichtinger W: Environmental factors and fertility. Hum Reprod 6:1170–1175, 1991.
15. Fink G: Gonadotropin secretion and its control. In Knobil E, Neill J (eds): The Physiology of Reproduction. New York, Raven, 1988, pp 349–377.
16. Florack EIM, Zielhuis GA, Pellegrino JEMC, Rolland R: Occupational physical activity and the occurrence of spontaneous abortion. Int J Epidemiol 22:878–884, 1993.
17. Gardner JM, Herz DE: Working and poor in 1990. Monthly Labor Review 20–28, December 1992.
18. Gaylor DW: Comparison of teratogenic and carcinogenic risks. Reg Toxicol Pharmacol 10:138–143, 1989.
19. Giacoia GP: Reproductive hazards in the workplace. Obstet Gynecol Surv 47:679–687, 1992.
20. Goldhaber MK, Rolen MR, Hiatt RA: The risk of miscarriage and birth defects among women who use visual display terminals during pregnancy. Am J Ind Med 13:695–706, 1988.
21. Goulet L, Theriault G: Stillbirth and chemical exposure of pregnant workers. Scand J Work Environ Health 17:25–31, 1991.
22. Gray RH, Corn M, Cohen R, et al: Final Report. The Johns Hopkins University Retrospective and Prospective Studies of Reproductive Health Among IBM Employees in Semiconductor Manufacturing. Baltimore, May 1993.
23. Hardin BD: Reproductive toxicity of the glycol ethers. Toxicology 27:91–102, 1993.
24. Hatch M: Introduction: Biological assessments in female reproductive toxicology. Environ Health Perspect 74:55–56, 1987.
25. Hooper K, LaDou J, Rosenbaum JS, Book SA: Regulation of priority carcinogens and reproductive or developmental toxicants. Am J Ind Med 22:793–808, 1992.
26. Joffe M: Detection of agents causing genetic or reproductive damage. Br J Ind Med 49:1–4, 1992.
27. Juutilainen J, Matilainen P, Saarikoski S, et al: Early pregnancy loss and exposure to 50-Hz magnetic fields. Bioelectromagnetics 14:229–236, 1993.
28. Keleher KC: Occupational health: How work environments can affect reproductive capacity and outcome. Nurse Pract 16:23–37, 1991.
29. Klebanoff MA, Shiono PH, Rhoads GG: Spontaneous and induced abortion among resident physicians. JAMA 265:2821–2825, 1991.
30. Koeter HBWM: Relevance of parameters related to fertility and reproduction in toxicity testing. Am J Ind Med 4:81–86, 1983.
31. Kotch JB, Ossler CC, Howze DC: A policy analysis of the problem of the reproductive health of women in the workplace. J Public Health Policy 5:213–227, 1984.
32. Kupfer D: Effects of pesticides and related compounds on steroid metabolism and function. Crit Rev Toxicol 4:83, 1975.
33. Lindbohm M-L, Hietanen M, Kyyronen P, et al: Magnetic fields of video display terminals and spontaneous abortion. Am J Epidemiol 136:1041–1051, 1992.
34. Lindbohm M-L, Taskinen H, Sallmen M, Hemminki K: Spontaneous abortions among women exposed to organic solvents. Am J Ind Med 17:449–463, 1990.
35. Lindbohm M-L, Sallmen M, Anttila A, et al: Paternal occupational lead exposure and spontaneous abortion. Scand J Work Environ Health 17:95–103, 1991.
36. Mamelle N, Laumon B, Lazar P: Prematurity and occupational activity during pregnancy. Am J Epidemiol 119:309–322, 1984.

37. Mattison DR, Thomford PJ: The mechanisms of action of reproductive toxicants. In Working P (ed): Toxicology of the Male and Female Reproductive Systems. New York, Hemisphere, 1989, pp 101–129.

38. McDonald AD, Armstrong B, Cherry NM, et al: Spontaneous abortion and occupation. J Occup Med 28:1232–1238, 1986.

39. McDonald AD, McDonald JC, Armstrong B, et al: Occupation and pregnancy outcome. Br J Ind Med 44:521–526, 1987.

40. McDonald AD, McDonald JC, Armstrong B, et al: Work with visual display units in pregnancy. Br J Ind Med 45:509–515, 1988.

41. Meisenheimer JR: How do immigrants fare in the US labor market. Monthly Labor Review 3–19, December 1992.

42. Messite J, Welch LS: An overview: Occupational health and women workers. Women and Work: An Ann Rev 2:21–44, 1987.

43. Moss N, Carver K: Pregnant women at work: Sociodemographic perspectives. Am J Ind Med 23:541–557, 1993.

44. National Center for Health Statistics: Advance report of maternal and infant health data from the birth certification. Vital Health Stat 42(suppl 2); 1990.

45. National Institute for Occupational Safety and Health: Criteria for a recommended standard: Occupational exposure to ethylene glycol monomethyl ether, ethylene glycol monoethyl ether, and their acetates. Cincinnati, NIOSH, 1991, US Dept of Health and Human Services publication NIOSH 91-119.

46. Nelson L, Kenen R, Klitzman S: Turning Things Around: A Women's Occupational and Environmental Health Resource Guide. Washington, DC, National Women's Health Network, 1990.

47. Ng TP, Foo SC, Yoong T: Menstrual function in workers exposed to toluene. Br J Ind Med 49:799–803, 1992.

48. Nurminen T, Kurppa K: Office employment, work with video display terminals and course of pregnancy. Scand J Work Environ Health 14:293–298, 1988.

49. Nurminen T, Lusa S, Ilmarinen J, Kurppa K: Physical work load, fetal development and course of pregnancy. Scand J Work Environ Health 15:404–414, 1989.

50. Olshan AF, Faustman EM: Male-mediated developmental toxicity. Reprod Toxicol 7:191–202, 1993.

51. Ouellet-Hellstrom R, Stewart WF: Miscarriages among female physical therapists who report using radio- and microwave-frequency electromagnetic radiation. Am J Epidemiol 138:775–786, 1993.

52. Ratcliffe JM, Schrader SM, Clapp DE, et al: Semen quality in workers exposed to 2-ethoxyethanol. Br J Ind Med 46:399–406, 1989.

53. Restrepo M, Munoz N, Day NE, et al: Prevalence of adverse reproductive outcomes in a population occupationally exposed to pesticides in Colombia. Scand J Work Environ Health 16:232–238, 1990.

54. Roman E, Beral V, Pelerin M, Hermon C: Spontaneous abortion and work with visual display units. Br J Ind Med 49:507–512, 1992.

55. Rosenman KD, Anderson HA, Selikoff IJ, et al: Spermatogenesis in men exposed to polybrominated biphenyl (PBB). Fertil Steril 32:209–213, 1979.

56. Rowland AS, Baird DD, Weinberg CR, et al: Reduced fertility among women employed as dental assistants exposed to high levels of nitrous oxide. N Engl J Med 327:993–997, 1992.

57. Sallmen M, Lindbohm ML, Anttila A, et al: Paternal occupational lead exposure and congenital malformations. J Epidemiol Community Health 46:519–522, 1992.

58. Saurel-Cubizolles MJ, Job-Spira N, Estryn-Behar M: Ectopic pregnancy and occupational exposure to antineoplastic drugs. Lancet 341:1169–1171, 1993.

59. Savitz DA, Whelan EA, Rowland AS, Kleckner RC: Maternal employment and reproductive risk factors. Am J Epidemiol 132:933–945, 1990.

60. Schaumburg I, Olsen J: Time to pregnancy among Danish pharmacy assistants. Scand J Work Environ Health 15:222–226, 1989.

61. Schenker MB, Samuels SJ, Perkins C, et al: Prospective surveillance of semen quality in the workplace. J Occup Med 30:336–344, 1988.

62. Schnorr TM, Grajewski BA, Hornung RW, et al: Video display terminals and the risk of spontaneous abortion. N Engl J Med 324:727–733, 1991.

63. Schrag SD, Dixon L: Occupational exposures associated with male reproductive dysfunction. Ann Rev Pharmacol Toxicol 25:567–592, 1985.

64. Sciarra JJ: Reproductive health: A global perspective. Am J Obstet Gynecol 168:1649–1653, 1993.

65. Selevan SG, Lindbohm M-L, Hornung RW, Hemminki K: A study of occupational exposure to antineoplastic drugs and fetal loss in nurses. N Engl J Med 313:1173–1178, 1985.

66. Sullivan FM: The European Community classification of chemicals for reproductive toxicity. Toxicol Lett 64/65:183–189, 1992.

67. Swan SH, Beaumont JJ, Hammond SK, et al: Historical cohort study of spontaneous abortion in semiconductor fabrication workers: Agent level analysis [unpublished manuscript].

68. Taskinen H: Prevention of reproductive health hazards at work. Scand J Work Environ Health 18(suppl 2):27–29, 1992.

69. Taskinen H, Anttila A, Lindbohm M-L, et al: Spontaneous abortions and congenital malformations among the wives of men occupationally exposed to organic solvents. Scand J Work Environ Health 15:345–352, 1989.

70. US General Accounting Office: Reproductive and Developmental Toxicants. Washington, DC, US General Accounting Office, October 1991.

71. Veulemans H, Steeno O, Masschelein R, Groeseneken D: Exposure to ethylene glycol ethers and spermatogenic disorders in man: A case-control study. Br J Ind Med 50:71–78, 1993.

72. Welch LS, Schrader SM, Turner TW, Cullen MR: Effects of exposure to ethylene glycol ethers on shipyard painters: II. Male reproduction. Am J Ind Med 14:509–526, 1988.

73. Wertheimer N, Leeper E: Fetal loss associated with two seasonal sources of electromagnetic field exposure. Am J Epidemiol 129:220–224, 1989.

74. Wertheimer N, Leeper E: Possible effects of electric blankets and heated waterbeds on fetal development. Bioelectromagnetics 7:13–22, 1986.

75. Whorton D, Krauss RM, Marshall S, Milby TH: Infertility in male pesticide workers. Lancet 2:1259–1261, 1977.

76. Wilcox AJ: Early pregnancy. In Kiely M (ed): Reproductive and Perinatal Epidemiology. Boca Raton, FL, CRC, 1991, pp 63–75.

77. Windham GC, Shusterman D, Swan S, et al: Exposure to organic solvents and adverse pregnancy outcome. Am J Ind Med 20:241–259, 1991.

78. Windham GC, Fenster L, Swan SH, Neutra R: Use of video display terminals during pregnancy and the risk of spontaneous abortion, low birthweight, or intrauterine growth retardation. Am J Ind Med 18:675–688, 1990.

79. Zielhuis GA, Gijsen R, van der Gulden JWJ: Menstrual disorders among dry cleaning workers. Scand J Work Environ Health 15:238, 1989.

MARI S. GOLUB, PhD
GERALD F. CHERNOFF, PhD

ISSUES IN REGULATORY PROTECTION OF REPRODUCTIVE HEALTH IN THE WORKPLACE

From the Reproductive and Cancer
 Hazard Assessment Section
Office of Environmental Health
 Hazard Assessment
California Environmental
 Protection Agency
Sacramento, California

Reprint requests to:
Mari S. Golub, PhD
Reproductive and Cancer Hazard
 Assessment Section
Office of Environmental Health
 Hazard Assessment
California Environmental
 Protection Agency
601 N. Seventh Street
Sacramento, CA 95814

Opinions expressed in this chapter
are those of the authors and do not
necessarily represent the position
of the California Environmental Protection Agency.

Ten years ago, adverse reproductive outcomes were termed "the occupational health issue of the 1980s."[51] Today it is clear that this issue was not resolved within the decade and has remained a major area of effort in regulatory programs designed to protect worker health. Lead, video display terminals (VDTs), solvents (glycol ethers in particular), and ethylene oxide have been toxic agents of particular concern in occupational settings over the past several years. As reproductive toxicity of pesticide residues has gained more public attention in connection with environmental contamination, the need to protect farm workers from these effects has become an issue.[28]

This chapter reviews the provisions of federal laws protecting reproductive health in the workplace and presents information on some recent actions at the federal level that seek to enhance this protection. In addition, two innovative regulatory programs administered by the state of California that directly address reproductive toxicity issues are described.

FEDERAL REGULATIONS PROTECTING REPRODUCTIVE HEALTH

The Occupational Safety and Health Act

Congressional action has resulted in three federal acts that are intended to control reproductive as well as other toxicity in the workplace. The first of these is the Occupational Safety and

Health Act enacted in 1970 to ensure, when possible, safe and healthful conditions in the workplace.[39] This act provides a mechanism for establishing and enforcing health-protective, permissible exposure limits (PELs) in the workplace. Individual states can establish different PELs as long as they are more protective than the federal levels.

According to the act, the National Institute for Occupational Safety and Health (NIOSH), which is part of the Centers for Disease Control, serves as the scientific arm responsible for developing data used in setting standards for workplace exposures. The adoption and enforcement of standards is the province of a second agency, the Occupational and Safety Health Administration (OSHA). In practice, the majority of OSHA's PELs are based on threshold limit values (TLVs) developed by the American Conference of Governmental Industrial Hygienists (ACGIH) and not on recommendations of NIOSH. Since TLVs are often based on unpublished data that are unavailable for public review, their use in establishing PELs has been criticized.[8,35] Of greatest concern from a scientific point of view is the lack of standardized guidelines or protocols for reviewing the data used to establish PELs. In spite of these limitations, PELs have been developed for some chemicals based on reproductive endpoints. Examples include dibromochloropropane (DBCP), ethylene oxide, and lead.

The Toxic Substances Control Act

In 1976, Congress enacted the Toxic Substances Control Act (TSCA) to protect the public health and environment from the production, use, and disposition of toxic substances.[40] The act, which specifically excludes pesticides, food additives, and nuclear material, provides the United States Environmental Protection Agency (EPA) with a mechanism for regulating commercial chemicals manufactured or imported into the United States.

The TSCA process begins with the identification and inventory of chemicals manufactured or imported into the United States. Data from toxicologic testing, including reproduction and development, may be requested, as well as reports of adverse reactions. For new chemicals, a review of data is required prior to entry of the substance into the marketplace. Chemicals that are found to pose a significant health risk can then be subject to regulation. The regulatory action can range from a prohibition on the manufacturing, processing, or distribution of the chemical, to limitations on the amount and conditions of use, or a requirement for a warning label. To date, the implementation of TSCA has resulted in very limited regulation based on reproductive endpoints, the one exception being the proposed regulation of two glycol ethers.[32] This can, in part, be attributed to the fact that reproductive and developmental toxicity tests are not specifically mandated under the act.

The Federal Insecticide, Fungicide, and Rodenticide Act

The Federal Insecticide, Fungicide, and Rodenticide Act (FIFRA) was enacted in 1982 to specifically address concerns regarding the health effects of pesticides.[41] The act provides the EPA with a mechanism for registering pesticides for use in the United States along with the setting of a tolerance or legal limit of use.

Central to FIFRA is the requirement for the manufacturer or registrant to provide data from a battery of prescribed studies. These include a multigeneration study usually conducted in rats, and two teratology studies, most often conducted in rats and rabbits. The testing protocols and requirements for data presentation are specified, thereby providing standardized results that can be compared across studies. Based on the results of the testing data, the EPA can set conditions of use and require specific warning language on the product label. Enforcement is carried out by the individual states.

FIFRA suffers from several potential and real limitations. Testing is conducted only on the active ingredients in the pesticide and excludes the inert ingredients that may make up more than 80% of the product. More importantly, the act grandfathered products that were in use prior to establishment of the testing requirements, thereby eliminating the requirement for studies on the majority of pesticides currently in use. A 1988 amendment to the act addressed this concern to a limited degree by creating lists of grandfathered pesticides for which there were concerns. There is also a process for conducting special reviews when data indicate that a pesticide may pose a health threat such as reproductive toxicity. This type of action resulted in the banning of Dinosep from the marketplace.

RECENT ADVANCES AT THE FEDERAL LEVEL

In addition to consideration of individual agents within existing programs, specialized policies and regulatory programs are being developed to address more general concerns about reproductive toxicity.[3] Particularly worthy of note at the federal level are the development of new animal test protocols for regulatory screening, establishment of guidelines for reproductive risk assessment, the fate of OSHA's PELs for glycol ethers, the report of the General Accounting Office (GAO) on reproductive toxicity, and the Supreme Court ruling concerning fetal protection policies.

Changes in Animal Screening Studies for Reproductive Toxicology

Many reproductive toxicants in the workplace are recognized by alert physicians or occupational health professionals. In addition, basic research in toxicology sometimes identifies these properties. However, the routine process established for identifying reproductive toxicity is standardized animal toxicology experiments that are required by FIFRA for registration of pesticides[42,44] and that have been carried over to other regulatory arenas. As mentioned above, two types of animal studies are usually required under current guidelines: a developmental toxicity study and a multigeneration study.

The developmental toxicity study, sometimes called the "teratology" study, was first required for use in 1979. Female breeders are administered different doses of the test agent during organogenesis and the early fetal period. Pregnant females are killed prior to term, and fetuses are examined for viability, malformation, and growth retardation.

Recently, developmental neurotoxicity testing guidelines have been provided for evaluating damage to the nervous system in offspring.[46] The study design calls for neurobehavioral and neurohistopathologic examination of offspring in the postnatal period. The developmental neurotoxicity guidelines offer an opportunity to go beyond traditional measures of mortality, malformation, and growth to look at functional abnormalities in offspring exposed to toxicants during development. Concern about well-known toxicants such as lead, mercury, and polychlorinated biphenyls (PCBs) is based primarily on their effects on mental development in children. Yet there has been no standardized way to examine the potential for agents to produce this type of effect. The developmental neurotoxicity guidelines attempt to fill this gap. In the future, evaluation of effects of developmental toxicants on function of the immune, endocrine, cardiovascular, pulmonary, and other systems may become more routine. Such determinations add an important dimension of security to standards that protect the pregnant worker.

The second required study is the multigeneration study, which yields information on male and female reproductive toxicity. Male and female breeders are administered the test agent prior to and during a period of cohabitation. Their offspring, the F1 generation, continue to receive the test agent after weaning and are subsequently mated to produce an F2 generation. All breeders are evaluated for fertility indices, pregnancy outcomes, and offspring growth and survival.

Recently, an alternative protocol for the multigeneration study, the reproductive assessment by continuous breeding (RACB) protocol,[27] has been put forward. In this protocol, the original breeders produce five consecutive litters, each litter being removed from the mother at birth so that breeding is continuous. The fifth litter serves as an F1 generation and is allowed to mature and reproduce.

The RACB protocol provides a relatively efficient approach to determining whether reproductive toxicity involves male and/or female breeders after the effects on mating pairs has been determined. To do this, a crossover mating (between males and females in exposed and unexposed groups) is included in the design of the study. The RACB also includes measures of sperm that make it possible to better integrate animal and human data on male reproductive toxicity. Studies have shown that the RACB is as effective as the current multigeneration study but is somewhat more sensitive and less expensive.[27] Routine use of this protocol would help in the screening of a series of related compounds for reproductive toxicity. For example, the RACB has recently been used to evaluate a series of glycol ethers[3,15,52] and phthalate esters.[14]

Reproductive Endpoints in Risk Assessment

An effort has been made to more fully use information on reproductive toxicity in the framework of the risk assessment process. In order to do this it is necessary to provide guidelines that define reproductive toxicity, describe how data should be evaluated, and provide procedures for determining safe exposure levels for various purposes, including for use in occupational settings.[17] Much of this work has been undertaken and advanced to consensus status, but much is still in process or the subject of controversy.

Risk assessment is the scientific determination of whether a substance is dangerous to health and how dangerous it is. Risk is the probability that any individual will suffer an adverse consequence as a result of exposure to a toxicant. Risk assessment is carried out primarily by scientists in government and industry and is also a specialized area in academia.

In a landmark document, the National Research Council[29] drew the distinction between risk assessment and risk management that has provided a structure for integrating science, policy, and regulatory practice. Risk assessment determines the risk; risk management seeks to minimize it in specific situations. These two processes are considered to work at their best when they are conducted independently. The EPA has assumed a leadership role in using this methodology and now relies on risk assessment in its programs regulating air and water contamination, hazardous waste, and pesticides. But the principles or risk assessment are now widely shared by worker and consumer protection programs. Cancer has been the endpoint driving most environmental risk assessments. However, more attention is being directed to noncancer endpoints, such as reproductive and developmental toxicity, neurotoxicity and immunotoxicity.[26]

The significance of risk assessment guidelines for reproductive toxicity is that they are designed to provide a uniform approach to evaluating reproductive toxicity and to establishing safe exposure levels (reference doses, no significant risk levels, permissible exposure limits) for regulatory purposes. Research findings will make their way into regulations governing exposure much more readily with such guidelines in place. Guidelines also ensure that a large number of agents can be considered in a standardized manner once basic principles of assessment have been established and accepted.

The EPA has taken the lead at the federal level in developing risk assessment guideline documents. In order to meet various programmatic needs, the EPA established an interagency working group to provide guidelines for developmental toxicity risk assessment. This group contained representatives of Food and Drug Administration, OSHA, the Consumer Products Safety Commission, and the EPA. A draft of the guidelines was published for public comment in the Federal Register in 1986[44] and was finalized after public comment in 1990.[43] The timeline for this project—1984–1990—reflects the difficulty of achieving a national standard in this area. State government[4] and private groups[16,24] also developed guidance documents in this area between 1990 and 1992, but many of the same basic principles are expressed in all of the documents.

Under the developmental toxicity risk assessment guidelines, both human and animal data are reviewed, with human data being given precedence. Standardized animal screening study designs, as described above, provide much of the data typically reviewed, but data from clinical medicine, epidemiologic studies, and basic research are also reviewed when available. Basic research can provide particularly critical information about the mechanism of action of the agent, which is useful in integrating other results. Standards for determining quality of a study and interpreting study endpoints are included in the guidelines. A "weight of evidence" approach to decision-making is used rather than a "critical study" approach.

Developmental toxicity is considered to be induced and manifested any time from birth to sexual maturity, although effects due to exposure during pregnancy and evaluations at the time of birth (birth defects) receive the most attention. A specialized topic for developmental toxicity is the issue of whether effects in the fetus are secondary to toxicity in the maternal system that results in a disruption of the pregnancy. If this is the case, protection of the worker in occupational settings should result in protection of the fetus. Thus, this is an important determination.

The EPA also has undertaken a project to establish guidelines for male and female reproductive toxicity.[47,48] Draft guidelines were issued in 1988, and a revision based on comments received was released in 1994.[49] State government and private groups have also developed guidelines in this area.[17,25]

A major unresolved issue concerns which endpoints measured in male and female reproductive toxicity are considered to represent adverse effects. The definition of reproductive toxicity grows unclear in several instances, primarily when changes in the reproductive system are encountered but are not known to result in infertility. For instance, are lowered sperm counts a valid index of reproductive toxicity, although the animals/men are still fertile? Is libido, or willingness to mate in animals, a valid reflection of reproductive toxicity? Can altered menstrual cycles be used as a basis for regulating exposures? In many cases, an index that is not in itself adverse will be taken as an early indicator or biomarker of reproductive toxicity.[30] However, a final determination of valid reproductive toxicity endpoints still awaits consensus.

Other issues relevant to both reproductive and developmental toxicity risk assessment are currently under active debate. These include whether agents should be classified as to the extent of certainty that they are hazardous (as with the International Agency for Research on Cancer [IARC] and EPA carcinogen categories), whether potency values can be derived to compare agents,[11] and what approach should be taken for determination of safe exposure levels.[21] For instance, approaches to mathematical modeling of dose-response data have been developed that allow determination of doses that produce particular incidences of adverse effects (i.e., 1%, 5%, 10%).[1]

As indicated above, developmental toxicity, or hazards to the developing fetus, infant, and child, is usually considered distinct from male and female reproductive toxicity, which are also distinguished from one another. In practice, however, data in these various areas are generally reviewed and evaluated together because much of the same data is relevant. For instance, human population exposures to environmental toxicants usually occur simultaneously to both members of a "couple." Also, as described above, the standard paradigm for regulatory testing, the multigeneration study, fails to distinguish male and female reproductive toxicity of "mating pairs." However, in the occupational setting the distinction is nevertheless helpful in determining who should be protected: all workers, male or female workers, or pregnant workers. Thus, refinements of testing and risk assessment procedures that help distinguish male, female, and developmental toxicity are valuable for those concerned with protecting workers.

PELs for Glycol Ethers

In occupational settings, assessment of risk and determination of safe exposure levels preceded the development of a formal federal risk assessment process. As described above, the Occupational Safety and Health Act of 1970 established OSHA, mandating that it establish and revise PELs for the workplace. In 1972 OSHA adopted about 400 exposure limits based on the ACGIH's 1968 threshold limit values as "national concensus standards" as specified under the law. Subsequently, the legislation required OSHA to generate, rather than adopt, PELs, and it required that they be supported by substantial scientific evidence. About 20 such standards were issued from 1972 to 1989; only one of these (DBCP) was based on reproductive toxicity.

Evidence of reproductive toxicity of glycol ethers began to appear in the early 1970s at about the same time that OSHA was established. At intervals NIOSH reviewed this information and published reports. In addition, field studies of appropriate worker groups were conducted. Recommended Exposure Levels (RELs) were also established by NIOSH. However, the PEL of 25 ppm for methyl cellosolve and ethoxyethanol, which was derived by ACGIH based on hematological endpoints, remained in effect.

In 1987, OSHA began developing new PELs for some glycol ethers based on reproductive toxicity. At about the same time, OSHA published an advanced notice of proposed rulemaking for Air Contaminant Standards as part of an initiative to significantly speed up issuance of new standards.[13] More than 400 values were prepared as part of the program. The glycol ether PELs, however, were not updated as part of this process due to the already ongoing activity in this area.

When OSHA published its final Air Contaminant Standards rule in the Federal Register in 1989 a number of lawsuits were filed by labor and industry representatives. Although several cases were settled, the entire rule was rejected in court in 1992 in connection with one of the lawsuits. The ruling was based partially on a failure to provide full analysis and documentation (e.g., risk assessment) on the health effects of all the agents involved in the rule, and, in particular, for lack of dose response assessment for "non-carcinogens." Meanwhile, further studies in worker populations, sponsored primarily by industry, have continued to implicate glycol ethers in adverse reproductive outcomes,[37] as documented elsewhere in this volume. A proposed rule directed specifically at glycol ethers has been published by OSHA[31] and has undergone public review. The PELs, based on NIOSH recommended standards, are 0.1 ppm for methoxyethanol and methoxyethanol acetate and 0.5 ppm for ethoxyethanol and ethoxyethanol acetate. It is hoped that these glycol ether PELs will be enacted in the near future. However, the time course of revision of PELs to reflect advances in information on reproductive toxicity remains discouraging.

The GAO Report on Reproductive Toxicants

Concern about reproductive toxicants led Congress to examine the effectiveness of federal regulatory control of environmental reproductive and developmental toxicants. In October 1991, the GAO, the investigative arm of Congress, issued a report titled "Reproductive and Developmental Toxicants: Regulatory Actions Provide Uncertain Protection."[50] The report was based on two surveys. The first survey was of scientific experts in developmental and reproductive toxicity and generated a list of 30 reproductive/developmental toxicants of greatest concern (Table 1). This list was then used as a basis of a survey of a number of federal agencies, including OSHA. The agencies were asked whether "bans, standards, and guidelines" for these chemicals that they had enacted were protective of reproductive effects.

Respondents at OSHA judged that 33% of 21 regulatory actions on these chemicals were protective. They reported using reproductive and developmental data in 43% of these actions. The GAO report pointed out that TLVs for seven of the agents were adopted from the 1968 ACGIH guidelines and had not subsequently been updated. Further, the GAO recommended that there be a limited time during which regulations adopted from outside authorities can be "maintained in lieu of federal decisions."

In the report, queried agencies frequently cited programmatic decisions for failure to regulate reproductive toxicants; however, the GAO suggested an active pattern of neglect of the relevant data. Also, while regulatory gaps were an identified problem, lack of rigorous risk assessment methods was also a concern.[12]

The GAO report and the generation of a specific list of agents has stimulated a great deal of reconsideration among federal government agencies. In addition, the scientific community, which was involved through generation of the list, has become more cognizant of the gap between scientific data and regulatory action.

Scientific Issues in Legal Actions on Fetal Protection Policies

An issue carried over from the 1980s[2] is the resolution of lawsuits concerning fetal protection policies. This debate has been carried forward largely in connection with the fetal protection policy of Johnson Controls, Inc.

TABLE 1. Chemicals of Concern as Reproductive and Developmental Toxicants[50]

Agent of Concern	Effect of Concern
Alcohol (ethyl alcohol)	Developmental, male
Arsenic	Developmental
Cadmium	Developmental, male
Carbon disulfide	Developmental, female, male
Carbon monoxide	Developmental
Chlordecone	Developmental, female, male
Chloroprene	Male
DDT	Developmental, female
DBCP	Female, male
DES	Developmental, female
Ethylene dibromide	Female, male
EGEE	Developmental, female, male
EGME	Female, male
Ethylene oxide	Female, male
Gossypol	Male
Hexachlorobenzene	Developmental, female
Lead	Developmental, female, male
Lithium	Developmental
Mercury	Developmental, female, male
Mirex	Female
Nicotine	Developmental
PBBs	Developmental, female
PCBs	Developmental, female
2,4,5-T	Developmental
TCDD	Developmental, female
Tobacco smoke[4]	Developmental, male
Toluene	Developmental, female
Vinyl chloride	Developmental, female, male
Vitamin A	Developmental
Warfarin	Developmental

Fetal protection policies can be seen as originating in Civil Rights legislation of 1964, which first introduced large numbers of women into jobs previously held exclusively by men and considered hazardous. Sex discrimination was explicitly forbidden under Title VII of the act, and pregnancy was specifically addressed in an amendment to Title VII, the Pregnancy Discrimination Act. However, larger companies and industries frequently established policies to protect women, especially pregnant women, in these jobs and sometimes to exclude or limit their participation as a way of preventing adverse reproductive outcomes. OSHA, labor unions, and the courts were seldom supportive of such policies. For instance, in 1978 OSHA promulgated its Lead Standard, which held that women should not be excluded from jobs involving lead exposure as had been recommended by the Lead Industries Association.

However, it was recognized that limitations on women could legitimately be placed under the "bona fide occupational qualification defense" if the work could not be performed adequately by women or pregnant women without unreasonable burden on the employer. One such potential unreasonable burden was susceptibility to tort liability for damage to the fetus, since liability was limited under Workers Compensation only for the worker and not for the fetus. Numerous legal challenges to fetal protection policies have centered on the issue of equal employment opportunity versus reproductive health hazards.[7] However, the issue has more broadly stimulated debate on institutional sexism[33] and the moral responsibility of employers to protect unborn children.[1a]

The fetal protection policy of Johnson Controls was first promulgated in 1982, challenged in court by the United Auto Workers (UAW) in 1984, upheld in two appellate courts (1988 and 1989), and finally ruled unconstitutional by the Supreme Court in 1991. The policy excluded women capable of bearing children from working in jobs involving the manufacture of lead batteries in which their blood lead level might rise above 30 μg/dL. Legal issues involved sex discrimination and civil rights of pregnant women and tort liability of employers for fetuses of workers. The Supreme Court decision did not rule that all fetal protection policies violate civil rights statutes but rather that certain aspects of the Johnson policy were unconstitutional. Thus, this decision will discourage but does not eliminate such policies. Further, this decision is currently relevant only within the U.S.; court systems of other countries have not reached similar decisions.[20]

Discussion of these cases in scientific fora has raised other issues such as the scientific definition of relative susceptibility and possible paternally mediated fetal effects.[10] In general, the commonly accepted premise that damage to the fetus is mediated exclusively by maternal exposure and that the fetus is more sensitive to toxic effects than its parents was not seen as based on scientific evidence but rather on the general moral/ethical standards. In addition, the point was taken that men's reproductive capabilities should be protected as vigorously as women's although this has not traditionally been a prominent concern. Also, the possibility that damage to the fetus could be mediated by toxicant exposure of the father was vigorously discussed. Thus, there is now an increased focus on male reproductive toxicity and possible mediation of effects on the fetus by exposure of the father.[18] These are currently active but controversial areas of interest in animal toxicology as well.

CALIFORNIA REGULATIONS PROTECTING REPRODUCTIVE HEALTH

The Birth Defects Prevention Act

In response to what was perceived as a failure on the part of the federal government to provide adequate health protection, California enacted two laws. The first, the Birth Defects Prevention Act, also known as SB950, was passed in 1984 in response to the grandfathered pesticides of FIFRA.[5] The act established a priority list of 200 pesticidal active ingredients for which data gaps must be filled within a specified amount of time. The testing requirements are similar to FIFRA, including prescribed multigenerational and teratology studies. The data from these studies are evaluated and reviewed by the Department of Pesticide Regulation of the California Environmental Protection Agency, which can then impose regulatory and labeling requirements. In cases in which an active ingredient is shown to cause a significant health hazard, mitigation requirements may be prescribed to minimize occupational and public exposures. In cases in which mitigation cannot provide a safe exposure level, the registrant may decide to withdraw the pesticide from the California market. While those responsible for enforcing this act have been criticized for not complying with the established time lines for review,[23] the act has resulted in the withdrawal of 37 pesticides.

Proposition 65

Unlike SB950 and the federal acts discussed above, California's Safe Drinking Water and Toxic Enforcement Act of 1986,[6] also known as Proposition 65, was not a product of legislation but rather an initiative of the people. Frustrated with the legislative process and reacting to what was perceived as a failure on the part of state and federal agencies to provide adequate health information and protection from hazardous chemicals, citizens petitioned for placement of the act on California's general election ballot in November 1986. Since the act did not have the benefit of legislative discussion and negotiations or lobbying efforts by interested parties, it is not surprising that a considerable amount of controversy surrounded both the election campaign and the early implementation of the law.[34] Opponents from industry and agriculture, as well as almost every newspaper in the state, claimed the measure to be extreme and unnecessary. The argument was put forth that existing laws were sufficient to protect the citizens of the state. It was predicted that the act would result in the listing and unnecessary regulation of thousands of chemicals, an avalanche of citizen enforcement suits that would create a lawyer's paradise, excessive warnings that would result in public confusion, and migration of businesses out of the state to avoid the threat of litigation and cost of conforming to the act. On the other side, proponents hailed the act as a revolutionary move toward a preventive strategy in the management of carcinogens and developmental and reproductive toxicants. They claimed that the number of listed chemicals would be small and that the public would benefit from knowing which chemicals have the potential to cause cancer, birth defects, and reproductive harm.[22] The act was passed by voters.

The premise of the proposition is that known carcinogens and developmental and reproductive toxicants (DARTs) will be identified through scientific decision-making and that the findings will be used to implement a public policy in which (1) citizens are informed when they are being exposed to significant levels of these agents; (2) the state's sources of drinking water are protected from contamination by these identified chemicals; and (3) the public is empowered to enforce this policy.

The major provisions of Proposition 65 address the listing of chemicals, warnings of exposure, prohibition of discharge, and enforcement options. They have been reported in detail elsewhere.[9,22,38] Briefly, the governor of California is required to publish at least once each year a list of those chemicals known to the state of California to cause cancer or reproductive toxicity. Twelve months after a chemical is placed on the list, any person who in the course of doing business knowingly and intentionally exposes any individual to significant levels of that chemical must first give a clear and reasonable warning. A warning is not required (1) if it is an exposure for which federal law governs warning in a manner that preempts state authority, (2) when the person responsible can show the exposure will pose "no significant risk" for carcinogens, or (3) when there will be no observable developmental or reproductive effect assuming 1000 times the level of the exposure in question. The act also states that 20 months after a chemical is placed on the list, no person in the course of doing business shall knowingly discharge or release a significant amount of the chemical into any present or potential source of drinking water. Failure to comply with the warning requirement or the discharge prohibition can result in a civil enforcement action initiated by either a public agency such as the state attorney general's office or any private citizen. Penalties may be up to $2,500 per day per violation, and successful actions by a private citizen entitle the citizen to receive 25% of the penalties. Businesses with fewer than 10 employees, government agencies, and public drinking water supply operations are not subject to the act.

To date, California's Proposition 65 list contains 140 developmental, 11 female reproductive, and 17 male reproductive toxicants. Four mechanisms for listing have been employed. The first mechanism, a minimum listing requirement, was mandated by specific language in the act. At a minimum, the list was required to contain substances identified by reference to California Labor Code Sections 6382 (b) (1) and 6382 (d). The second mechanism provides for the listing of chemicals that in the opinion of the "state's qualified experts" have been clearly shown through scientifically valid testing according to generally accepted principles to cause cancer or reproductive toxicity. A third mechanism is the use of formal pronouncements by authoritative bodies recognized by the "state's qualified experts." Recognized authoritative bodies are EPA, the U.S. Food and Drug Administration, IARC, the National Toxicology Program, and NIOSH. In the fourth mechanism, a chemical that is formally required to be labeled or identified as a carcinogen or reproductive toxicant by a state or federal agency is eligible for automatic listing.

Under Proposition 65, listed chemicals are subject to warning requirement and discharge prohibition unless it can be shown that exposures meet specified exemption criteria. For DARTs, the act set the specific exemption standard as an exposure that will have no observable effect assuming exposure at one thousand times the level in question. In practice, this means applying a 1000-fold uncertainty factor to the most appropriate no observed adverse effect level from experimental data.

According to Proposition 65, the party responsible for an exposure or discharge bears the burden of proving that the exposure or discharge meets the exemption criteria. To assist the enforcement and regulated communities, the state has developed regulatory levels for 3 DARTs and has several more in progress. Exposures below these levels do not require a warning, nor are they subject to the discharge prohibition. These levels are intended to provide guidance in the form of "bright lines" or "safe harbors" for businesses subject to the provisions of the proposition, and they do not preclude the use of an alternative level that can be demonstrated by its user as being scientifically valid.

For the regulatory community, Proposition 65 has had a tangible benefit in that it provides a clear mechanism for identifying chemicals of concern, an efficient process for establishing acceptable levels of exposure to these chemicals, and an effective means of enforcement. For most environmental statutes such as the Toxic Substances Control Act, enforcement cannot proceed until a regulatory limit has been set by the EPA. This provides an incentive for delaying the setting of the levels to avoid compliance. With Proposition 65, once a chemical is listed there is an incentive to determine levels that are in compliance with the statute. It is not required that the state set a level; businesses can develop their own. However, without a set number, the level of concern drops to any detectable amount.

Proposition 65 also represents an additional tool by which California regulatory agencies can enforce violations of related laws. For example, a food product with elevated amounts of lead from its packaging can be found to be in violation of food safety laws and, in the absence of a warning, also in violation of Proposition 65. Illegal discharge of hazardous waste resulting in the contamination of drinking water sources may be prosecuted under both hazardous waste laws and Proposition 65.

While it is obvious that Proposition 65 has had clear and meaningful benefits, it would be unfair to say that there have been no problems. The implementation of the act is still evolving, and there are definite areas of concern that deserve attention. Most notable are the concerns with the method of warning. At present, there is a lively debate about the potential for inappropriate warnings, warnings for which there is no significant level of exposure or for which no exposure exists at all. Also of concern is whether the type of information given in the warnings is sufficiently clear. This is especially true for DARTs, where the time of exposure may be the critical factor in determining an adverse outcome. These concerns are currently under consideration and should be resolved in the near future.

Concern also has been raised that the 1000-fold uncertainty factor applied to DARTs is unscientific and overly conservative.[36] While this is undoubtedly true for some agents, for others a greater uncertainty factor may be appropriate. Since the 1000-fold factor is in the language of the act, any change will require a two-thirds majority vote in both houses of the California legislature. This is unlikely in the near future since any legislation to amend must "further the purposes" of the act.

While Proposition 65 applies to worker as well as consumer exposure, OSHA requirements for providing toxicity information are usually considered to meet the requirements of the proposition for warning of workers. However, the public empowerment provision is a major new dimension in occupational settings. To date, two lawsuits have been initiated by employees against employers under the provisions of Proposition 65. The first (Thomas v. Berkeley Horticultural Nursery, Alameda County Superior Court) dealt with exposure to asbestos during removal of insulation and was settled out of court. The second (Badenell v. Zurn Industries, San Obispo Superior Court) deals with failure to warn of workplace exposures to lead. This case has been referred to federal court and is ongoing. Depending on the outcome of these cases, lawsuits by employees against employers under Proposition 65 may become more common.

REFERENCES

1. Beck BD, Conolly RB, Dourson ML, et al: Improvements in quantitative noncancer risk assessment. Fundam Appl Toxicol 20:1–14, 1993.
1a. Becker ME: Can employers exclude women to protect children? JAMA 264:2113–2117, 1990.
2. Bertin JE: Reproduction, women, and the workplace: Legal issues. Occup Med State Art Rev 1:497–507, 1986.
3. Bossert NL, Reel JR, Lawton AD, et al: Reproductive toxicity of triethylene glycol and its diacetate and dimethyl ether derivatives in a continuous breeding protocol in Swiss CD-1 mice. Fundam Appl Toxicol 18:602–608, 1992.
4. California Environmental Protection Agency, Reproductive and Cancer Hazard Assessment Section: Draft guidelines for assessing developmental and reproductive toxicity: Hazard identification and dose-response assessment. Sacramento, April 1991.
5. California Food and Agriculture Code: Section 13121 et seq., 1984.
6. California Health and Safety Code: Section 25249.5, et seq., 1986.
7. California Policy Seminar: Reproductive Health Hazards in the Workplace: Policy Options for California. University of California, Berkeley, 1992.
8. Castleman BI, Ziem G: Corporate influence on threshold limit values. Am J Ind Med 13:531–559, 1988.
9. Chernoff GF, Book SA: Reproductive hazard evaluation and risk assessment under California's Proposition 65. In Neubert D, Kavlock RJ, Merker H-J, Klein J (eds): Risk Assessment of Prenatally-Induced Adverse Health Effects. Heidelberg, Germany, Springer-Verlag, 1992, pp 181–190.
10. Colie C: Male mediated teratogenesis. Reprod Toxicol 7:3–9, 1993.

11. Fabro S, Shull G, Brown NA: The relative teratogenic index and teratogenic potency: Proposed components of developmental toxicity risk assessment. Teratogenesis Carcinog Mutagen 2:61–76, 1982.

12. Gibbons A: Reproductive toxicity: Regs slow to change. Science 254:25, 1991.

13. Gordon C (OSHA attorney): Personal communication, 1992.

14. Heindel JJ, Gulati DK, Mounce RC, et al: Reproductive toxicity of three phthalic acid esters in a continuous breeding protocol. Fundam Appl Toxicol 12:508–518, 1989.

15. Heindel JJ, Gulati DK, Russell VS, et al: Assessment of ethylene glycol monobutyl and monophenyl ether reproductive toxicity using a continuous breeding protocol in Swiss CD-1 mice. Fundam Appl Toxicol 17:270–279, 1990.

16. Institute for Evaluating Health Risks: An evaluation process for determining human reproductive and developmental toxicity of agents. Washington, DC, March 5, 1992.

17. Infante PF, Tsongas TA: Occupational reproductive hazards: Necessary steps to prevention. Am J Ind Med 4:383–390, 1983.

18. Joffe M: Male- and female-mediated reproductive effects of occupation: The use of questionnaire methods. J Occup Med 31:974–979, 1989.

19. [Reference deleted.]

20. Johnston KJ, Jamieson GG, Wright S: Reproductive and developmental hazards and employment policies. Br J Ind Med 49:85–94, 1992.

21. Kimmel CA, Wellington DG, Farland W, et al: Overview of a workshop on quantitative models for developmental toxicity risk assessment. Environ Health Perspect 79:209–215, 1989.

22. Kizer KW, Warriner TE, Book SA: Sound science in the implementation of public policy: A case report on California's Proposition 65. JAMA 260:951–955, 1988.

23. Lightstone R: Pesticide poisoning and environmental data in California. Rural California Report 2, 1990.

24. Mattison DR, Hanson J, Kochhar DM, Rao KS: Criteria for identifying and listing substances known to cause developmental toxicity under California's Proposition 65. Reprod Toxicol 3:3–12, 1990.

25. Mattison DR, Working PK, Blazak WF, et al: Criteria for identifying and listing substances known to cause reproductive toxicity under California's Proposition 65. Reprod Toxicol 4:163–175, 1990.

26. McMaster SB: Developmental toxicity, reproductive toxicity and neurotoxicity as regulatory endpoints. Toxicol Lett 68:225–230, 1993.

27. Morrissey RE, Lamb JC IV, Morris RW, et al: Results and evaluations of 48 continuous breeding reproduction studies conducted in mice. Fundam Appl Toxicol 13:747–777, 1989.

28. Moses M: Pesticide related health problems in farm workers. Assoc Am Occup Health Nurs J 37:115–130, 1989.

29. National Research Council: Risk assessment in the federal government: Managing the process. Washington, DC, National Academy Press, 1983.

30. National Research Council: Biologic markers in reproductive toxicology. Washington, DC, National Academy Press, 1989.

31. Occupational Safety and Health Administration: Occupational exposure to 2-methoxyethanol, 2-methoxyethanol and their acetates (glycol ethers); Proposed rule. 29 CFR Part 1910, Federal Register 58:15526–15632, 1993.

32. Office of Technology Assessment: Reproductive health hazards in the workplace. Washington, DC, Congress of the United States, 1985.

33. Pollitt K: A new assault on feminism. The Nation, March 26, 1990.

34. Roberts L: A corrosive fight over California's toxic law. Science 243:306–309, 1989.

35. Robinson JC, Paxman DG, Rappaport SM: Implications of OSHA's reliance on TLVs in developing the Air Contaminant Standard. Am J Ind Med 19:3–13, 1991.

36. Russell C: Proposition 65 California's controversial gift. APF Reporter 12:33–38, 1989.

37. Schenker M: Epidemiologic study of reproductive and other health effects among workers employed in the manufacture of semiconductors. Final report to the Semiconductor Industry Association, San Jose, CA, December 1992.

38. Totten G: Controversial Proposition 65 provokes industry outrage, 'quiet compliance' as it marks second anniversary as law. Chem Reg Report, 169–174, May 1989.

39. United States Code 29: Sections 651–678, 1976.

40. United States Code 15: Sections 2601–2629, 1976.

41. United States Code 7: Sections 136–136y, 1982.

42. United States Environmental Protection Agency, Office of Pesticides and Toxic Substances: Health effects test guidelines. Washington, DC, EPA document 560/6-82-001, 1982.

43. United States Environmental Protection Agency: Guidelines for developmental toxicity risk assessment. Federal Register 65:234, 63798–63826, 1990.
44. United States Environmental Protection Agency: Guidelines for health assessment of suspect development toxicants. Federal Register 51:34027–34040, 1986.
45. United States Environmental Protection Agency: In vivo reproductive and mutagenicity test. Springfield, VA, US Dept of Commerce, 1982.
46. United States Environmental Protection Agency: Pesticide assessment guidelines—subdivision F—Hazard Evaluation: Human and domestic animals. Addendum 10: Neurotoxicity. Series 83-A, Developmental Neurotoxicity Study. EPA document 540/090910123. Springfield, VA, US Dept of Commerce, National Toxicology Information Service, 1991.
47. United States Environmental Protection Agency: Proposed guidelines for assessing female reproductive risk. Federal Register 53:24835–24847, October 1988.
48. United States Environmental Protection Agency: Proposed guidelines for assessing male reproductive risk. Federal Register 53:24850–24869, October 1988.
49. United States Environmental Protection Agency: Draft guidelines for reproductive toxicity risk assessment. EPA/600/AP-94/001, 1994.
50. United States General Accounting Office: Reproductive and developmental toxicants: Regulatory actions provide uncertain protection. Washington, DC, GAO publication PEMD-92-3.
51. Whorton MD: Adverse reproductive outcomes: The occupational health issue of the 1980s. Am J Public Health 73:15–16, 1983.
52. Williams J, Reel JR, George JD, Lamb JC IV: Reproductive effects of diethylene glycol and diethylene glycol monoethyl ether in Swiss CD-1 mice assessed by a continuous breeding protocol. Fundam Appl Toxicol 14:622–635, 1990.

JAMES W. OVERSTREET, MD, PhD

CLINICAL APPROACH TO MALE REPRODUCTIVE PROBLEMS

From the Division of Reproductive
  Biology and Medicine
Department of Obstetrics and
  Gynecology
    and
Institute of Toxicology and
  Environmental Health
University of California
Davis, California

Reprint requests to:
James W. Overstreet, MD, PhD
Institute of Toxicology and
  Environmental Health
University of California
Davis, CA 95616

Supported by the National Institute
of Environmental Health Sciences
Superfund Basic Research Program (P42ES04699) and by NIEHS
(P01ES06198).

Although there has been rapid progress in our understanding of human reproductive biology and in the treatment of infertility, our knowledge of male reproductive problems has not kept pace with other advances in the field. There also has been a realization that occupational and environmental factors may play an important role in human infertility[108] and that the male may be particularly vulnerable to these adverse effects.[96] Nevertheless, identification of these reproductive hazards has proven to be difficult.

One of the problems that arises in the assessment of reproductive hazards in the workplace is identification of men who may have work-related infertility or subfertility. The problem is twofold. First, the clinical definition of infertility requires a period of unsuccessful attempts to conceive a pregnancy. Most diagnostic and prognostic criteria for clinical evaluation of the subfertile male are based on the assumption of such a history. For this reason, the clinical assessment of men who have "abnormal" laboratory findings (e.g., low sperm counts) but who have not attempted to achieve a pregnancy is problematic. Second, many risk factors for male subfertility have been recognized, including a number of lifestyle variables, but few have been clearly proven to cause infertility. This uncertainty will cause difficulty in establishing a cause-effect relationship between suspected occupational hazards and male reproductive problems. Nevertheless, when suspected reproductive hazards are identified, a thorough clinical evaluation of the male is indicated. This chapter will review the clinical and laboratory approach that is currently recommended for such an evaluation.

CLINICAL EVALUATION OF THE MALE

The Sequence and Pace of the Clinical Evaluation

An infertility evaluation involves the couple. Therefore, both the male and female should be evaluated. The work-up of the two partners should be coordinated, and communication between clinicians should be maintained throughout the period of evaluation. Evaluation of the male is managed by a clinical andrologist who may be trained as a urologist or endocrinologist (a subspecialty of internal medicine); less frequently, a gynecologist may take this role. In clinical practice, the obstetrician-gynecologist who carries out the work-up of the female is frequently the primary physician for the couple. At the time the work-up of the female is initiated, a semen evaluation should be obtained for the male. If the semen evaluation is unquestionably normal, there may be no further evaluation of the male until the work-up of the female is completed. However, if the semen evaluation is abnormal or marginal, an immediate clinical evaluation is indicated. Such an evaluation begins with a history and physical examination, evaluation of semen, and evaluation of endocrine function. Based on the findings of the initial work-up, additional clinical diagnostic tests and/or specialized laboratory tests may be indicated. If the semen evaluation was initially normal, the work-up of the male may be deferred until the work-up of the female is completed, usually 4 to 6 months after the first visit to the clinic. The diagnosis of unexplained infertility is never appropriate until the male, as well as the female, has been completely evaluated and found to be normal.

History

The history should be focused not only on the reproductive and sexual histories, but also on the occupational, social, medical, and surgical histories. As discussed previously, the duration of infertility is of critical importance in assessing impairment of reproductive function. The fecundability or monthly probability of conception is approximately 25% in healthy young couples who do not practice birth control.[58] The reproductive and sexual history should establish the frequency of coitus, use of birth control, and the likelihood that unprotected intercourse has taken place during the fertile period of the menstrual cycle. These considerations are most important when the duration of infertility is relatively short (12 months or less). Longer durations of infertility in sexually active couples are less likely to be related to the frequency and timing of coitus.

The physician should develop a clear understanding of the couple's knowledge of human reproduction and sexuality. The normal functions of erection, ejaculation, intromission, and orgasm should be discussed and evaluated. For couples who are actively trying to conceive, the strategy for becoming pregnant should be discussed in detail. There is considerable self-help literature on this subject, and many technical aids are commercially available. Couples can easily delay or prevent conception by misunderstanding or misapplying this knowledge and technology. When more than one physician is involved in the management of the couple's evaluation, it is also important that consistent instructions are given and that no misinformation is imparted. Couples using home ovulation predictor kits and/or basal body temperature charts should be instructed in their interpretation for detecting ovulation. Intercourse should begin before the expected day of ovulation and should occur at approximately 2-day intervals. This timing takes advantage of the fact that sperm survive for at least 2 days in the female reproductive tract.[40] Because the sperm reserves of the male require at least 2 days for replenishment,[2] intercourse or ejaculation that is more frequent than every 2 days may decrease the male's fertility. The use of artificial lubricants such as K-Y jelly, Lubifax, Surgilub and Keri-lotion during coitus may interfere with fertility because they decrease sperm motility.[9,38]

The reproductive history of both partners is important because it may indicate preexisting fertility or infertility. Such information should include a history of all previous pregnancies and their outcomes. The reproductive histories of previous partners should be elicited. Any previous infertility evaluation or treatment of the couple or their previous partners also should be discussed.

The medical and surgical history should begin with childhood. The time of puberty may be precocious in conditions such as congenital adrenal hyperplasia[22] or may be delayed in cases of hypothalamic-pituitary dysfunction.[103] Cryptorchidism, whether unilateral or bilateral, is a risk factor for subsequent infertility,[62] and this risk is not eliminated following orchidopexy.[61] Childhood surgery in the inguinal region, such as herniorrhaphy, may result in blockage of the vas deferens. Childhood bladder surgery may have included Y-V plasty of the bladder neck at the time of ureteral implantation.[100] This procedure may result in subsequent retrograde ejaculation. Mumps infection prior to puberty has no effect on subsequent testicular function, but mumps orchitis occurs unilaterally in 30% of men infected after puberty, and 10% may have bilateral orchitis.[112] Even in men with unilateral orchitis, the effect on fertility may be severe.

Medical problems such as diabetes mellitus may affect erection and ejaculation.[42] Thyroid disease,[53] liver disease,[111] and renal disease[45] have been associated with male infertility. Infertility patients may have a history of malignant disease. The radiation and/or chemotherapy required to cure malignancies often has profound side effects on fertility.[95] Cancer surgery also involves significant risk of subsequent infertility. Retroperitoneal lymph node dissection may result in damage to the sympathetic nerves and consequent failure of emission or ejaculation.[55]

Infection with tuberculosis or veneral diseases such as chlamydia and gonorrhea may result in blockage of the reproductive tract.[33] Transient effects on the testis may be induced by systemic infection, genitourinary infection, or any febrile illness. When there is a history of recent acute illness and the semen evaluation is abnormal, it is important to repeat the evaluation after approximately 74 days to allow for a new cycle of spermatogenesis.[2] The finding of normal semen on the repeat evaluation will indicate that there was a reversible effect of the illness on spermatogenesis.

In addition to occupational exposures that are discussed elsewhere in this volume, the medical history should include information on drugs or medications that could impair spermatogenesis. These drugs include cimetidine,[110] salfasalazine,[59] and nitrofuradantoin.[77] Recreational drugs such as ethanol,[109] tobacco,[30] marijuana,[54] and cocaine[6] may also be toxic to the testes, as may androgenic steroids.[46]

Physical Examination

The physical examination of the subfertile male is focused on the gonads, the male reproductive tract, the accessory sex glands, and the external genitalia. The body habitus should be consistent with normal virilization, including body fat and body hair distribution, as well as absence of gynecomastia. Other aspects of the general physical examination are also relevant to the infertility work-up. For example, hepatomegaly may be observed in association with abnormalities of hormone metabolism, pituitary tumors may cause abnormal visual fields, and thyromegaly may be detected during evaluation of the head and neck.

The anatomy of the penis should be examined for its adequacy to deposit semen in the vagina. Abnormal penile curvature or abnormal location of the urethral meatus should be noted. Testicular size should be measured in two dimensions, and testicular consistency should be assessed by palpation. Testicular volume can be estimated with an orchiodometer. The normal adult testis ranges in length from 4.1–5.5 cm and in width from 2.1–3.2 cm; the testicular volume ranges from 20–30 mL.[97] Damage to the seminiferous tubules usually results in abnormally small testes, because these structures account for the great majority of the testicular volume. When the tubules are damaged prior to puberty the testes are characteristically firm; postpubertal damage typically results in soft testes.[67]

The epididymis should be palpated for signs of obstruction including evidence of dilation, nodularity, or cystic changes. The vas deferens should be palpated bilaterally. The pampiniform venous plexus should be palpated for evidence of dilation, which is called a varicocele. Varicoceles are classified as grade 1 if palpable with Valsalva maneuver, grade 2 if palpable without the Valsalva maneuver, and grade 3 if visible through the scrotal wall. Varicocele is a common finding among subfertile men. The role of varicocele in infertility is controversial, but most experts agree that this condition may contribute to infertility in some men, and when found in combination with abnormal semen, varicoceles should be surgically corrected.[47]

A rectal examination should be performed to assess the prostate, which should be firm and nontender. A large and/or tender prostate may indicate infection. The seminal vesicles are not normally palpable during the rectal examination, and when they are found, there may be an obstruction in the ejaculatory duct.

SEMEN EVALUATION

The semen evaluation is the most basic laboratory test for clinical assessment of the subfertile male. This single test provides information on sperm production by the testes, patency of the reproductive tract, activity of the accessory glands, and capability for ejaculation. Nevertheless, interpretation of semen parameters may be complicated. Abnormal findings in the absence of a history of infertility may be difficult to interpret. Conversely, the absence of abnormal findings does not necessarily imply that a male is fertile, because traditional measurements of semen quality are superficial and the laboratory methodology on which they are based is often subjective and lacking in standardization.

Specimen Collection and General Semen Properties

Semen evaluation usually requires analysis of several specimens because of the significant day-to-day variability in semen parameters.[83] Sperm numbers in semen may vary with the season and may be reduced during the summer months.[60] As previously discussed, febrile illness and lifestyle factors also may induce transient semen abnormalities. Therefore, a single abnormal semen evaluation is never sufficient to establish that male reproductive function is impaired. Because sexual activity also affects semen quality,[102] there should be a period of sexual abstinence before evaluation; 48–72 hours is usually recommended.[79]

The semen is usually collected by masturbation, and it is important that the laboratory supply the specimen container because many plastics are spermicidal. Semen-collection condoms also can be used,[123] but contraceptive condoms are not appropriate because they are spermicidal. When semen samples are collected at home and transported to the laboratory, there is a risk that sperm motility will be affected after collection because of temperature fluctuations or aging during transportation. Many clinical laboratories provide a private room for semen collection to avoid these potential artifacts.[79]

The semen evaluation may vary in complexity depending on the capabilities of the laboratory and the requirements of the clinician. The basic parameters that are measured describe sperm numbers, sperm motility, and sperm morphology in the ejaculate. These parameters may be assessed subjectively or they may be measured objectively. Measurements can be made manually or with computer-aided sperm analysis (CASA) systems. Modern andrology laboratories are now equipped to measure most semen parameters automatically, but the technology has still not developed to the point where all semen analyses can be routinely automated.[24]

The semen should be evaluated as soon as possible after ejaculation and always within 1 hour of collection. The semen is evaluated in several steps. Semen volume is measured to the nearest 0.1 mL using a serological pipette. The specimen as a whole is examined for color and odor. It is normally opaque and gray-white in color; yellow, pink, or red coloration is abnormal. Abnormal odors such as urine or putrefaction should be noted. Semen pH is typically 7.2–7.8,[29] but abnormalities of pH have not been associated with infertility.

Most semen is coagulated (clot-like) immediately after ejaculation and liquifies gradually during the next 15–30 minutes. Specimens that have not fully liquified within 1 hour are considered abnormal.[84] Semen coagulation should be distinguished from semen viscosity, which is measured after liquifaction is complete. Semen viscosity can be measured on a subjective scale of 0 (water-like) to 4 (gel-like), or more objective methods can be used, such as measuring the rate at which drops are formed when the semen is allowed to flow from a 0.1-mL pipette.[29] Although high semen viscosity may interfere with some steps in the semen evaluation, there is no good evidence that this property of semen is directly related to infertility.

Microscopic Evaluation of Semen

SPERM MOTILITY

Following assessment of the general semen properties, the specimen is evaluated microscopically. Sperm motility is assessed with phase-contrast microscopy at 37°C. Visual assessment of percent motility is carried out by observing at least 200 sperm. A motile sperm is defined as any sperm with a moving flagellum, whether or not the sperm is progressing. Forward progression, as assessed visually, is often rated for the sperm suspension as a whole. For example, on a scale of 1 to 4, a score of 1 indicates no sperm progression, a score of 2 indicates sluggish to fair progression, a score of 3 indicates good progression, and a score of 4 indicates highly vigorous progression. In other protocols, the percentage of progressive sperm is counted in addition to the overall percent motility,[115] or a "sperm drive" based on sperm velocity may be calculated to quantify sperm progression.[122]

Although percent motility can be counted accurately using visual methods, these methods are probably not satisfactory for obtaining information on sperm motility beyond the presence or absence of progressive sperm. However, quantitative data on sperm motility and progression can now be obtained with a variety of CASA instruments (see below).

SPERM CONCENTRATION

Sperm concentration is determined on a aliquot of the semen, which is diluted with a fixative or a spermicidal solution. Sperm numbers may be counted manually with a hemocytometer[115] or with a specialized counting chamber such as a Makler Chamber[66] or Microcell Chamber.[79] CASA instruments can be used to measure sperm concentrations automatically, but errors are encountered when there are low or high sperm concentrations, significant sperm agglutination, or large amounts of seminal debris.[24]

OTHER MICROSCOPIC OBSERVATIONS

Other microscopic observations of the semen include assessments of sperm agglutination[74] and observations of epithelial cells, protozoa, bacteria, and round cells. Round cells may include both leukocytes and prematurely exfoliated, immature germ cells. The identity of round cells cannot be determined with phase contrast microscopy, but most round cells can be classified on a stained seminal smear (see below).

SPERM MORPHOLOGY

Sperm morphology is evaluated on seminal smears that are prepared at the time of semen evaluation and subsequently stained. The Papanicolaou stain is commonly used, but a variety of stains, including special stains, can be employed.[115] Sperm morphology is usually assessed with bright-field, oil immersion optics, and the most important parameter in the clinical assessment of sperm morphology is the percentage of "normal" spermatozoa in the sample.

There is controversy regarding the definition of a morphologically normal sperm. Most clinical laboratories use some version of the World Health Organization (WHO) criteria, which specify metric standards for the length and width of normal sperm heads.[115,116] More strict morphological criteria can be used to define a normal sperm, with the result that more sperm are excluded from the normal category because of subtle abnormalities in head shape and staining properties.[68] Thus, semen from fertile men may have as few as 14% normal sperm by strict criteria,[68] in comparison with a 50% cutoff when the WHO criteria of 1987[116] are used. The situation has been further confused by the 1992 revisions of the WHO criteria, which include new metric standards and more strict requirements for a normal classification; the recommended cutoff for normal sperm morphology with this new protocol is 30%.[115]

Most morphology classification protocols assign abnormal sperm to separate categories on the basis of their structural abnormalities. It should not be surprising that there is also no consensus on the definitions of abnormal sperm types. Although metric standards for classification of abnormal sperm have been proposed,[51] these standards have not been widely applied. Nevertheless, there are specific situations in which a knowledge of the types of abnormal sperm may be useful in the clinical assessment of subfertile males. Sperm with a "round-head defect" have agenesis of the acrosome and are nonfunctional cells. This condition appears to be congenital, and when present in all sperm, the abnormality leads to complete sterility.[121] Tapered sperm are found more frequently in the semen of infertile men if they have a varicocele,[76] and the presence of such sperm in the semen of men with varicocele may be an indication for varicocelectomy. Epididymal dysfunction may be suspected when there is coiling of the sperm tail or other flagellar abnormalities[89]; unfortunately, there is no specific therapy for such disorders.

EVALUATION OF ROUND CELLS IN SEMEN

The stained seminal smear also can be used to evaluate round cells, most of which are likely to be either leukocytes or immature germinal cells. Seminal granulocytes can be counted in a hemocytometer following peroxidase staining.[115] Polymorphonuclear leukocytes can be recognized on a Papanicolaou-stained smear on the basis of nuclear morphology, and their concentration in semen can be estimated from the ratio of leukocytes to sperm cells on the seminal smear.[79] Positive identification of round cells in semen can be made using special staining procedures with monoclonal antibodies to leukocyte antigens.[114] A leukocyte concentration greater than 10^6/mL is considered abnormal.[115]

Automated Semen Analysis

CASA instruments have the ability to make precise measurements of sperm concentration, percent motility, and sperm movement characteristics,[24] as well as to assess sperm morphology.[23] However, application of these instruments requires standardization of procedures and careful attention to quality control. Special protocols are required to analyze semen specimens with low sperm concentrations because misclassification of seminal debris in such specimens may lead to significant errors. In specimens with high sperm concentrations, sperm collisions lead to artifacts as a result of overlap in sperm trajectories, which the computer may erroneously interpret. Therefore, semen specimens with sperm concentrations of greater than 40×10^6 sperm per milliliter must be diluted prior to analysis. These limitations have restricted the application of CASA for routine clinical evaluations, and there is a significant risk that the instruments, when used improperly, may provide inaccurate data on sperm concentration and motility.[24] Similarly, instruments for automated sperm morphology assessments currently provide different results when the same sperm are analyzed,[107] because image processing hardware and classification algorithms have not been standardized.

Interpretation of Semen Parameters

The minimum standards for fertile semen have been derived from a number of large-scale clinical studies in which the results of semen analyses from fertile and infertile men were compared.[63,92,124] Unfortunately, when semen parameters have been used to predict fertility, the results have been disappointing. These studies have either found no parameter predictive of fertility[91] or that different parameters were predictive in different studies.[8,28,90] These studies were hampered by use of subjective methods of semen analysis and by reliance on a single semen evaluation for prediction of fertility. Nevertheless, the fact that most studies found one or more parameters of semen quality predictive of fertility is encouraging that more consistent results can be obtained if multiple evaluations are performed using objective laboratory methods.

In current clinical practice, semen parameters can only be used to classify semen into general categories such as "normal," "marginal" or "abnormal." The definitions of the categories are arbitrary, although they are based on existing clinical data. The normal range for semen volume is 2.0–5.0 mL (Table 1). Both large and small semen volumes are associated with male infertility.[26] Large semen volume may result in an abnormally low sperm concentration, even when total sperm output by the testes is adequate. Low semen volumes may be inadequate to buffer the vaginal acidity and could therefore result in rapid sperm immobilization in the vagina. When abnormal semen volumes contribute to infertility, these effects should be reflected in an abnormal postcoital test (see below). If the postcoital test is normal, abnormalities of semen volume are unlikely to have clinical significance.

The numbers of sperm in semen provide a quantitative assessment of the function of the germinal epithelium, and for this purpose the total sperm number per ejaculate (sperm concentration × semen volume) is an informative semen parameter. The cutoff point for normal sperm numbers per ejaculate is frequently set at 40 million sperm per milliliter[115] (40×10^6/mL). The sperm concentration in semen or the sperm count has a broad range of normal values, with a lower limit usually set at 20 million sperm per milliliter[65] (20×10^6/mL). There is clinical evidence that fertility is also impaired at high sperm concentrations,[36] but there is no biological explanation for this observation. Low sperm numbers in themselves may not be an important cause of infertility providing that the sperm have normal function. This conclusion is suggested by reports of fertile men with normal spermatogenesis but low sperm counts. Well-recognized examples of such men are those treated with contraceptive agents[5] and patients with hypogonadotropic hypogonadism who are treated with exogenous gonadotropins.[13] These clinical examples as well as experimental data[34,71,72] suggest that abnormal sperm function rather than insufficient sperm numbers is the probable cause of infertility in men with low sperm counts.

Sperm motility has been measured in large clinical studies of fertile and infertile men,[64,92,124] but the methodology in these older studies was subjective, and the results cannot be applied for interpretation of contemporary sperm movement characteristics. A lower limit for percentage of motile sperm in the range of 40–50% (see Table 1) is in general agreement with the recommendations of the older clinical studies. The existing clinical literature provides little guidance on parameters of normal sperm progression. Although CASA instruments can measure a variety of sperm movement parameters, the straight line velocity, or VSL, is considered to be the most robust parameter for clinical analysis of sperm progression in semen.[25] The cutoff point for normal sperm progression has been set provisionally at 25 μm/sec.[25] The other sperm movement characteristics that can be measured with CASA instruments are not yet used routinely for clinical evaluations.

TABLE 1.   Classification of Semen Quality

Semen Parameter	Normal Semen Quality	Marginal Semen Quality	Abnormal Semen Quality
Semen volume (mL)	2–5*	1–2	< 1
Sperm concentration (× 10^6/mL)	20–250*	10–20	< 10
Sperm motility (% motile)	> 50	40–50	< 40
Straight-line velocity (μm/sec)	> 25	20–25	< 20
Sperm morphology (% normal)	> 50†	40–50	< 40

* Values that exceed the upper range of normal may result in classification of the semen as marginal or abnormal.
† As assessed by the 1987 criteria of the World Health Organization[116]

As previously discussed, the normal values for sperm morphology depend on the protocol that is used for morphological assessment. In clinical practice, morphology assessment protocols seldom are rigorously applied, and variation in morphology results is considerable, both within and between technicians and laboratories.[4,27]

Parameters of sperm numbers, motility, and morphology are correlated with one another,[35,74,99] and for this reason multiplication of individual parameters (for example, semen volume × sperm concentration × % motility) is no more predictive of male fertility than single parameters alone.[90] In clinical practice, individual parameters are often used to assign patients to clinical categories.[15,79] In our institution, the following categories are used: (1) semen quality within normal limits, no evidence for infertility; (2) marginal semen quality, infertility is possible; and (3) abnormal semen quality, infertility is likely (see Table 1). Assignment of patients to prognostic categories requires clinical judgment because of the multiplicity of semen parameters and the normal variability in semen properties. When one or more semen parameters falls within an abnormal or marginal range of values (for example, marginal sperm motility), the patient usually is assigned to the corresponding clinical category (in this case, marginal semen quality). In general, the patient is assigned to the clinical category that reflects the poorest of the semen parameters recorded.

Depending on individual variability, a number of semen evaluations may be required to classify a patient. Even a normal semen evaluation should be confirmed by repeat evaluation. Patients with abnormal semen may have one or more paramters that are within the normal range of values. As previously discussed, men with low sperm concentrations but otherwise normal semen have a good prognosis for fertility. Isolated abnormalities of sperm motility can result from structural abnormalities of the sperm tail,[121] but the possibility of an artifact being induced by semen collection, transportation, or handling also should be considered. A finding of marginal or abnormal semen quality should lead to a complete clinical evaluation of the male. When the semen quality is marginal, complete evaluation of the female is also warranted because female factors also may be contributing to the couple's infertility.

SPECIALIZED LABORATORY TESTS ON SPERM

Semen evaluations that produce objective, quantitative data usually provide the clinician with a reliable impression of the male contribution to a couple's infertility. However, the clinical studies that correlate these modern semen parameters with fertility endpoints are still lacking. As a result, other specialized tests are often carried out on sperm to gain additional information on the likelihood of male fertility. These tests may be carried out in follow-up of abnormal results on the standard semen evaluation or they may be used following a normal semen evaluation to search for otherwise unrecognized abnormalities in male reproductive function. Unfortunately, these tests suffer from many of the same problems as the standard semen evaluation: insufficient standardization and lack of rigorous assessment in clinical studies.

Tests of Sperm Structures or Organelles

PLASMA MEMBRANE INTEGRITY

There are many approaches for assessing the integrity of the sperm plasma membrane. In general, these tests rely on the detection of a cytological stain that is too large to cross an intact plasma membrane. Sperm that exclude the stain are frequently referred to as "viable" sperm. Such viable sperm are not identical to motile sperm, and sperm with abnormalities of the flagellar structure[121] would be recognized with such methods as viable cells even though they are immotile. Many conventional stains can be used in sperm viability testing, such as eosin or trypan blue.[115] Fluorescent nuclear stains such as the Hoechst dye 33258 (H258) also have been widely applied to sperm.[19] Flow cytometry approaches have been developed for assessing sperm membranes, including dual fluorescent staining technology for simultaneous assessment of plasma membrane and mitochondrial membrane integrity.[31]

Another test of sperm viability is the hypoosmotic swelling (HOS) test.[122] This test evaluates whether sperm have intact membranes by assessing their ability to respond osmotically. In addition to membrane integrity, the HOS test appears to measure functions of the sperm membrane that are involved in the transport of water. Like other viability tests, HOS test results correlate relatively poorly with motility.[122] The test results are considered normal if more than 60% of the sperm tails swell in hypoosmotic medium, abnormal if less than 50% swell, and borderline if 50–60% swell.[122] Although the clinical data are not conclusive, many studies have reported this to be a useful test in assessing male fertility.[122]

ACROSOMAL INTEGRITY AND FUNCTION

The acrosome is an essential organelle of the sperm cell, and it functions in response to signals from the oocyte to enable sperm penetration of the oocyte investments and sperm fusion with the oolemma.[119] In rare fertility disorders, the acrosome may be missing from otherwise normally formed spermatozoa.[121] More often, acrosomal dysfunction is suspected as a cause of infertility.[82]

The acrosome can be evaluated with electron microscopy,[121] or cytological techniques can be used to visualize the acrosome with the light microscope. Conventional straining techniques,[105] fluoresceinated lectins,[19] and monoclonal antibodies[113] have been used. Because acrosomal loss may be a normal consequence of sperm death, most cytological approaches employ a second supravital stain to identify viable, acrosome-reacted sperm.[19,105]

Acrosomal function may be tested using bioassays such as tests of sperm-zona pellucida interaction or sperm penetration assays using zona-free hamster oocytes (see below). A variety of chemical and biological agonists of the acrosome reaction may be used to evaluate acrosomal function. These agonists include the calcium ionophore A23187,[21] human follicular fluid,[14] cumulus oophorus,[106] or disaggregated zona pellucida.[20] No cutoff points for infertility have been established with these acrosomal function tests, although biological reasoning and the limited data suggest that these tests can identify sperm populations with subnormal fertilizing capacity.

Bioassays of Sperm Function

These laboratory tests take advantage of complex biological materials to assess a number of integrated functions of the sperm cell. Because the basic cell biology of sperm function is often poorly understood, interpretation of the test results is only possible at the descriptive level. As bioassays, the tests have proven difficult to standardize or control for quality. Nevertheless, these tests will remain an important tool for assessing sperm function until they can be replaced with specific tests such as the tests of acrosomal function described previously.

SPERM-CERVICAL MUCUS INTERACTION

Tests of interaction between sperm and cervical mucus are usually performed in follow-up to an abnormal postcoital test and seek to determine the cause of sperm-cervical mucus incompatibility.[85] In general, the tests involve observations of sperm-cervical mucus interaction in vitro. A number of testing protocols have been proposed. Some involve observation of sperm-mucus interaction on a microscopy slide.[69] Others require measurements of sperm penetration into mucus-filled capillary tubes.[52,86] The sperm functions that are assessed in these tests primarily involve sperm motility, which is required both for entry into mucus and for progression in mucus,[32] and interactions between the sperm surface and the cervical mucus macromolecules that may impede sperm movement through the mucus.[81] One well-established abnormality of the sperm surface that is often revealed in tests of sperm-cervical mucus interaction is the presence of antisperm antibodies.[57] There are no widely accepted values for normal sperm-cervical mucus interaction tests. Because cervical mucus is a highly variable biological fluid, these tests must always be run with appropriate controls. It was once thought that bovine cervical mucus could be used as a more standardized substitute for human mucus. However, it is now recognized that bovine mucus cannot be substituted for human mucus in these assays.[115] These tests are most valuable when used in a cross-testing protocol.[83] In such a protocol semen and cervical mucus from the infertile couple are tested in a four-way comparison with normal semen and cervical mucus from fertile donors. The results of such cross-mucus penetration tests provide information on the sources of semen-mucus incompatibility: the semen, the cervical mucus, or both. The results of these tests point the direction for additional laboratory and/or clinical studies.

SPERM PENETRATION OF ZONA-FREE HAMSTER OOCYTES

The sperm penetration assay (SPA) arose from the observation that the zona pellucida is the primary block to interspecies fertilization for the golden hamster and that, when the zona is removed from hamster oocytes in the laboratory, sperm from virtually any species, including humans, can fuse with the plasma membrane of the oocyte and decondense in the ooplasm.[118] Because these are important steps in fertilization, there was great optimism that the SPA would be an incisive test of male fertility. Although these fertilization functions and the prerequisite steps of sperm capacitation and the acrosome reaction are measured by the SPA, a number of other important functions are not assessed with this assay, including sperm transport to the oocyte and sperm penetration of the oocyte investments.[41]

Standardization of the SPA in clinical laboratories has also proven to be difficult. In addition to the unavoidable variability inherent in a bioassay, the SPA has been complicated by innumerable variations involving media, incubation time, temperature, and additions of chemical and biological agents to modify sperm function in the assay.[93,120] In current practice, the SPA has less value in predicting male infertility than it has as a screening tool for assisted reproductive technology programs. In this context, the test results may be used to assess the likelihood for success of in vitro fertilization (IVF) and to suggest modifications of sperm preparation and IVF conditions, such as modification or supplementation of the culture media, for subfertile semen.[75]

SPERM-ZONA PELLUCIDA IINTERACTION

Tests of sperm-zona pellucida interaction are not widely available because they require zonae pellucidae of human oocytes, which are always in short supply.

These assays, like the SPA, are used to investigate sperm functions required for fertilization. In general, the results of zona pellucida assays provide information on sperm capacitation and the acrosome reaction, as well as specific functions such as sperm binding to the zona and sperm penetration through the zona. The specific functions measured are complementary to those measured in the SPA, and in some studies the assays have been used together as a mixed gamete assay.[82] As with the SPA, there are many variations of these assays, including whole frozen-stored zonae,[80] salt-stored zonae,[117] or hemi-zonae.[12] The clinical utility of the assays is primarily for prediction of success with IVF.[78]

Biochemical Tests of Sperm Functions

The seminal plasma is a highly complex biological fluid, and numerous biochemical tests have been employed to characterize its properties.[37] Because relatively little is known of the biological functions of the seminal fluid, these tests have little clinical utility. However, some components of the sperm cell can be measured biochemically and may have clinical relevance. Acrosin is one of the acrosomal enzymes that is thought to play a role in sperm penetration of the zona pellucida,[119] and concentrations of this enzyme have been found to differ in sperm samples from fertile and infertile men.[39,56,70] Adenosine triphosphate (ATP) also has been investigated as a marker for sperm fertility, but its clinical value is controversial.[50] The most promising biochemical test under current investigation is creatine phosphokinase (CK), whose isoform CK-M has been proposed as a biomarker of sperm maturation.[48,49]

Tests for Antisperm Antibodies

The need to test for antisperm antibodies may be indicated by historical risk factors or by results of preceding laboratory tests. Tests for antisperm antibodies should be included in the evaluation of any male before a diagnosis of unexplained infertility is reached. The development of antisperm antibodies in the male may be associated with disruption of the anatomical blood-testis barrier or blood-epididymal barrier.[43] Therefore, a history of conditions predisposing to breech of these barriers such as infection, genital trauma, obstruction, or surgery may warrant antisperm antibody testing. Sperm agglutination in semen may be caused by antibodies, and the report of vigorously motile, agglutinated sperm on the semen evaluation may indicate a need for antibody testing. Abnormalities of sperm-mucus interaction, including abnormal postcoital tests or abnormal sperm-cervical mucus penetration tests, also should be followed up with antibody testing.

Although many tests have been used for circulating antisperm antibodies, the value of this information is limited because there is relatively poor correspondence between antisperm antibodies in blood and semen.[44] Only antibodies that are actually attached to sperm are likely to impair their function, and for this reason the most informative tests for antisperm antibodies are those that assess sperm cells directly. The immunobead test (IBT)[11] and the radiolabeled immunoglobulin test[43] have this capability, but the IBT is used most commonly. For the IBT, sperm are mixed with beads that have been coated with Ig-class specific second antibodies. The sperm suspension is observed microscopically for agglutination of sperm and beads. The IBT results include the percentage of sperm binding beads, the region of the sperm involved (head, midpiece, tail), and the immunoglobulin class. The results are considered clinically significant by some investigators if 20% or more of sperm bind beads,[16] but others set this cutoff at 50%.[3,10] Some evidence exists that immunoglobulins of the IgA class may be more detrimental than those of IgG.[87] Head-associated antisperm antibodies are also thought to be more detrimental to fertility than are antibodies directed against the tip of the sperm tail.

EVALUATION OF THE ENDOCRINE SYSTEM

Abnormalities of the endocrine system are a relatively infrequent cause of male subfertility, but the endocrine evaluation is an important component of the male fertility evaluation. The baseline evaluation is aimed at assessment of the hypothalmic-pituitary-testicular axis and is accomplished by measurements of serum luteinizing hormone (LH), follicle-stimulating hormone (FSH), and testosterone. Failure of spermatogenesis is usually associated with an elevation of serum FSH because of pituitary release from the negative feedback of inhibin.[94] Elevated FSH levels in a patient with small atrophic testes and significant semen abnormalities usually indicate irreversible testicular damage. On the other hand, when normal FSH levels are associated with abnormal semen, the cause of infertility may involve posttesticular lesions such as epididymal obstruction. Because many abnormalities of spermatogenesis may occur without elevation of FSH, disorders of spermatogenesis cannot be distinguished from obstructive lesions when the endocrine evaluation is normal. In these cases, additional clinical investigation including testicular biopsy, scrotal exploration, and vasography may be indicated (see below). Low levels of LH, FSH, and testosterone may indicate hypogonadotropic hypogonadism, which may respond to therapy with exogenous gonadotropins.[101] In patients with hypogonadotropic hypogonadism, other pituitary hormones should be assessed. Measurements of prolactin and estradiol and tests of thyroid function are rarely indicated for male infertility patients.[67]

CLINICAL DIAGNOSTIC TESTS

Clinical diagnostic tests including testicular biopsy, vasography, and ultrasound evaluations are used to identify men with ductal obstruction that may be treated surgically. Although testicular biopsy provides the information for definitive diagnosis of testicular failure, the procedure is seldom necessary when the semen is markedly abnormal, the testes are atrophic, and the FSH levels are elevated. In cases with azoospermia or severely abnormal semen but a normal endocrine evaluation, a biopsy finding of active spermatogenesis may indicate surgically correctable obstruction of the reproductive tract.[98] However, when spermatogenesis is present but abnormal, the testicular biopsy usually does not provide specific information on the cause of spermatogenic dysfunction, nor does it contribute to the choice of therapy.[18]

Definitive information on the site of obstruction in the vas deferens, seminal vesicles, or ejaculatory ducts is obtained from vasography in which radioopaque contrast medium is instilled into the vas.[7] More recently, transrectal ultrasound has been used as a relatively noninvasive method to visualize the seminal vesicles and ejaculatory ducts for evidence of obstruction.[88] Blockage of the epididymis is determined by observation of dilated epididymal tubules at the time of scrotal exploration.

CONCLUSION

The approach for evaluation of male reproductive function follows a logical sequence of basic clinical evaluations and laboratory tests, which are followed by more specialized tests and procedures as indicated by the initial work-up. At the conclusion of this evaluation process, the physician will have substantial evidence with which to determine the contribution of the male to the couple's infertility. Information will be available on genetic, environmental, and lifestyle factors that may be associated with infertility. The site of reproductive dysfunction, whether the gonads, the endocrine system, or the male reproductive tract, will be known, and the prognosis for future fertility can be estimated. The tests of sperm function that are currently available enable the identification of many abnormalities of sperm physiology. This knowledge has led to a number of successful therapies based on in vitro technology[1] and manipulation of gametes.[17] Unfortunately, understanding of the causes of sperm dysfunction at the level of spermatogenesis is much more limited. As a result, the pathophysiology of most cases of male subfertility is unclear, and definitive therapy is also lacking. As our basic understanding of spermatogenesis improves, rapid application of this knowledge in the clinical setting can be anticipated.

REFERENCES

1. Acosta AA: Male factor in assisted reproduction. Infertil Reprod Med Clin North Am 3:487–503, 1992.
2. Amann RP: A critical review of methods for evaluation of spermatogenesis from seminal characteristics. J Androl 2:37–60, 1981.
3. Ayvaliotis B, Bronson R, Rosenfeld D, et al: Conception rates in couples where autoimmunity to sperm is detected. Fertil Steril 43:739–742, 1985.
4. Baker HWG, Clarke GN: Sperm morphology: Consistency of assessment of the same sperm by different observers. Clin Reprod Fertil 5:37–43, 1987.
5. Barfield A, Melo J, Coutinho E, et al: Pregnancies associated with sperm concentrations below 10 million/ml in clinical studies of a potential male contraceptive method, monthly depot medroxyprogesterone acetate and testosterone esters. Contraception 20:121 127, 1979.
6. Berul CI, Harclerode JE: Effects of cocaine hydrochloride on the male reproductive system. Life Sci 45:91, 1989.
7. Boreau J: Images of the Seminal Tracts. New York, Karger, 1974.
8. Bostofte E, Bagger P, Michael A, et al: Fertility prognosis for infertile men: Results of follow-up study of semen analysis in infertile men from two different populations evaluated by the Cox regression model. Fertil Steril 54:1100–1106, 1990.
9. Boyers SP, Corrales MD, Huszar G, et al: The effects of lubrin on sperm motility in vitro. Fertil Steril 47:882–884, 1987.
10. Bronson RA, Cooper GW, Rosenfeld DL: Autoimmunity to spermatozoa: Effect on sperm penetration of cervical mucus as reflected by postcoital testing. Fertil Steril 41:609–614, 1984.
11. Bronson RA, Cooper GW, Rosenfeld DL: Sperm antibodies: Their role in infertility. Fertil Steril 42:171–183, 1984.
12. Burkman LJ, Coddington CC, Franken DR, et al: The hemizona assay: Development of a diagnostic test for the binding of human spermatozoa to the human hemizona pellucida to predict fertilization potential. Fertil Steril 49:688–697, 1988.
13. Burris AS, Clark RV, Vantman DJ, et al: A low sperm concentration does not preclude fertility in men with isolated hypogonadotropic hypogonadism after gonadotropin therapy. Fertil Steril 50:343–347, 1988.
14. Calvo L, Vantman D, Banks SM, et al: Follicular fluid-induced acrosome reaction distinguishes a subgroup of men with unexplained infertility not identified by semen analysis. Fertil Steril 52:1048–1054, 1989.
15. Clark RV, Sherins RJ: Use of semen analysis in the evaluation of the infertile couple. In Santen RJ, Swerdloff RS (eds): Male Reproductive Dysfunction. New York, Marcel Dekker, 1986, pp 253–266.
16. Clarke GN, Elliott PJ, Smaila C: Detection of sperm antibodies in semen using the immunobead test: A survey of 813 consecutive patients. Am J Reprod Immunol Microbiol 7:118–123, 1985.
17. Cohen J, Talansky BE, Alikani M, Adler A: Micromanipulation of gametes. Infertil Reprod Med Clin North Am 3:505–524, 1992.
18. Colgan TJ, Dedard YC, Strawbridge HTG, et al: Reappraisal of the value of testicular biopsy in the investigation of infertility. Fertil Steril 33:56–60, 1980.

19. Cross NL, Morales P, Overstreet JW, Hanson FW: Two simple methods for detecting acrosome-reacted human sperm. Gamete Res 15:213–226, 1986.
20. Cross NL, Morales P, Overstreet JW, Hanson FW: Induction of acrosome reactions by the human zona pellucida. Biol Reprod 38:235–244, 1988.
21. Cummins JM, Pember SM, Jequier AM, et al: A test of the human sperm acrosome parameters. J Androl 12:98–103, 1991.
22. Cutfield RG, Bateman JM: Infertility caused by bilateral testicular masses secondary to congenital adrenal hyperplasia. Fertil Steril 40:809–814, 1983.
23. Davis RO, Bain DE, Siemers RJ, et al: Accuracy and precision of the Cellform-human automated sperm morphometry instrument. Fertil Steril 58:763–769, 1992.
24. Davis RO, Katz DF: Computer-aided sperm analysis: A critical review. In Centola GM, Ginsburg KA (eds): Evaluation and Treatment of the Infertile Male. Cambridge, England, Cambridge University Press, 1994 (in press).
25. Davis RO: The promise and pitfalls of computer-aided sperm analysis. Infertil Reprod Med Clin North Am 3:341–352, 1992.
26. Dubin L, Amelar RD: Etiologic factors in 1294 consecutive cases of male infertility. Fertil Steril 22:469–474, 1971.
27. Dunphy BC, Kay R, Barratt CLR, et al: Quality control during the conventional analysis of semen, an essential exercise. J Androl 10:378–385, 1986.
28. Dunphy BC, Neal LM, Cooke ID: The clinical value of conventional semen analysis. Fertil Steril 51:324–329, 1989.
29. Eliasson R: Analysis of semen. In Behrman SJ, Kistner RW (eds): Progress in Infertility. 2nd ed. Boston, Little, Brown & Co., 1975, pp 691–713.
30. Evans HJ, Fletcher J, Torranre M, et al: Sperm abnormalities and cigarette smoking. Lancet 1:627–629, 1981.
31. Evenson DP, Darzynkiewicz Z, Melamed MR: Simultaneous measurement by flow cytometry of sperm cell viability and mitochondrial membrane potential related to cell motility. J Histochem Cytochem 30:279–280, 1982.
32. Feneux D, Serres C, Jouannet P: Sliding spermatozoa: A dyskinesia responsible for human infertility? Fertil Steril 44:508–511, 1985.
33. Fowler JE: Genital tract infection. In Lipshultz LI, Howards SS (eds): Infertility in the Male. 2nd ed. St. Louis, Mosby, 1991, p 297.
34. Franken DR, Oehninger S, Burkman LJ, et al: The hemizona assay (HZA): A predictor of human sperm fertilizing potential in in vitro fertilization (IVF) treatment. J In Vitro Fert Embryo Transf 6:44–50, 1989.
35. Freund M: Interrelationships among the characteristics of human semen and factors affecting semen specimen quality. J Reprod Fertil 4:143–159, 1962.
36. Glezerman M, Bernstein D, Zakut CH, et al: Polyzoospermia—a definite pathological entity. Fertil Steril 38:605–608, 1982.
37. Glezerman MG, Bartoov B: Semen analysis. In Insler V, Lunenfeld B (eds): Infertility. New York, Churchill Livingstone, 1986, pp 243–271.
38. Goldenberg RL, White R: The effect of vaginal lubricants on sperm motility in vitro. Fertil Steril 26:872–873, 1975.
39. Goodpasture JC, Zavos PM, Cohen MR, et al: Relationship of human sperm acrosin and proacrosin to semen parameters. I. Comparison between symptomatic men of infertile couples and asymptomatic men, and between different split ejaculates. J Androl 3:151–156, 1982.
40. Gould JE, Overstreet JW, Hanson FW: Assessment of human sperm function after recovery from the female reproductive tract. Biol Reprod 31:888–894, 1984.
41. Gould JE, Overstreet JW, Yanagimachi H, et al: What functions of the sperm cell are measured by in vitro fertilization of zona-free hamster eggs? Fertil Steril 40:344–352, 1983.
42. Greene LF, Kelalis PO, Weeks RE: Retrograde ejaculation of semen due to diabetic neuropathy. J Urol 98:693–696, 1967.
43. Haas GG Jr: Immunologic male infertility. Infertil Reprod Med Clin North Am 3:413–427, 1992.
44. Hellstrom WJG, Overstreet JW, Samuels SJ, Lewis EL: The relationship of circulating antisperm antibodies to seminal antibodies in infertile men. J Urol 140:1039–1044, 1988.
45. Holdsworth S, Atkins RC, de Kretser DM: The pituitary-testicular axis in men with chronic renal failure. N Engl J Med 296:1245–1249, 1977.
46. Holma PK: Effects of an anabolic steroid on spermatogenesis. Contraception 15:151, 1977.
47. Howards SS: Varicocele. Infertil Reprod Med Clin North Am 3:429–441, 1992.

48. Huszar G, Vigue L, Corrales M: Sperm creatine kinase activity in fertile and infertile oligospermic men. J Androl 11:40–46, 1990.

49. Huszar G, Vigue L: Incomplete development of human spermatozoa is associated with increased creatine phosphokinase concentration and abnormal head morphology. Mol Reprod Dev 34:292–298, 1993.

50. Irvine DS, Aitkin RJ: The value of adenosine triphosphate (ATP) measurements in assessing the fertilizing ability of human spermatozoa. Fertil Steril 44:806–813, 1985.

51. Katz DF, Diel L, Overstreet JW: Differences in the movement of morphologically normal and abnormal human seminal spermatozoa. Biol Reprod 26:566–570, 1988.

52. Katz DF, Overstreet JW, Hanson FW: A new quantitative test for sperm penetration into cervical mucus. Fertil Steril 33:179–186, 1980.

53. Kidd GS, Glass AR, Vigersky RA: The hypothalamic-pituitary-testicular axis in thyrotoxicosis. J Clin Endocrinol Metab 48:798–802, 1979.

54. Kolodny RC, Masters WH, Kolodny RM, Toro G: Depression of plasma testosterone levels after chronic intensive marihuana use. N Engl J Med 290:872–874, 1974.

55. Kom C, Mulholland SG, Edson M: Etiology of infertility after retroperitoneal lymphadenectomy. U Urol 105:528–530, 1971.

56. Koukoulis G, Vantman D, Banks SM, et al: Low acrosin activity in a subgroup of men with idiopathic infertility does not correlate with sperm density, percent motility, curvilinear velocity, or linearity. Fertil Steril 52:120–127, 1989.

57. Kremer J, Jager J: The sperm-cervical mucus contact test: A preliminary report. Fertil Steril 27:335–340, 1976.

58. Leridon H: Human Fertility: The Basic Components. Chicago, University of Chicago Press, 1977.

59. Levi AJ, Fisher A, Hughes L, et al: Male infertility due to sulphasalazine. Lancet 2:276–278, 1979.

60. Levine RJ, Mathew RM, Chenault CB, et al: Differences in the quality of semen in outdoor workers during summer and winter. N Engl J Med 323:12–16, 1990.

61. Lipshultz LI, Caminos-Torres R, Greenspan CS, et al: Testicular function after orchidopexy for unilaterally undescended testes. N Engl J Med 295:11, 1976.

62. Lipshultz LI: Cryptorchidism in the subfertile male. Fertil Steril 27:609–620, 1976.

63. MacLeod J, Gold RZ: Semen quality in 1000 men of known fertility and 800 cases of infertile marriage. Fertil Steril 2:115–139, 1951.

64. MacLeod J, Gold RZ: The male factor in fertility and infertility. III. An analysis of motile activity in the spermatozoa of 1000 fertile men and 1000 men in infertile marriage. Fertil Steril 2:187–204, 1951.

65. MacLeod J, Wang Y: Male fertility potential in terms of semen quality: A review of the past, a study of the present. Fertil Steril 21:103–116, 1979.

66. Makler A: The improved ten-micrometer chamber for rapid sperm count and motility evaluation. Fertil Steril 33:337–338, 1980.

67. McClure RD: Endocrine investigation and therapy. Urol Clin North Am 14:471–488, 1987.

68. Menkveld R, Stander FSH, Lotze TJ, et al: The evaluation of morphological characteristics of human spermatozoa according to stricter criteria. Hum Reprod 5:586–592, 1990.

69. Moghissi KS: Cyclic changes of cervical mucus in normal and progestin-treated women. Fertil Steril 17:663–675, 1966.

70. Mohsenian M, Syner FN, Moghissi KS: A study of sperm acrosin in patients with unexplained infertility. Fertil Steril 37:223–229, 1982.

71. Morales P, Overstreet JW, Katz DF: Changes in human sperm motion during capacitation in vitro. J Reprod Fertil 83:119–128, 1988.

72. Morales P, Katz DF, Overstreet JW, et al: The relationship between the motility and morphology of spermatozoa in semen. J Androl 9:241–247, 1988.

73. Mortimer D, Templeton AA, Lenton EA, et al: Semen analysis parameters and their interrelationships in suspected infertile men. Arch Androl 8:165–171, 1982.

74. Mortimer D: The male factor in infertility: Semen analysis. Curr Probl Obstet Gynecol 8:1–81, 1985.

75. Muller CH: The andrology laboratory in an assisted reproductive technologies program. J Androl 13:349–360, 1992.

76. Naftulin BN, Samuels SJ, Hellstrom WJG, et al: Semen quality in varicocele patients is characterized by tapered sperm cells. Fertil Steril 56:149–151, 1991.

77. Nelson WD, Steinberger E: The effect of furadoxyl upon the testis of the rat. Anat Rec 112:367–368, 1952.

78. Oehninger S, Coddington CC, Scott R, et al: Hemizona assay: Assessment of sperm dysfunction and prediction of IVF outcome. Fertil Steril 51:665–670, 1989.

79. Overstreet JW, Davis RO, Katz DF: Semen evaluation. Infertil Reprod Med Clin North Am 3:329–340, 1992.
80. Overstreet JW, Hembree WC: Penetration of the zona pellucida of nonliving human oocytes by human spermatozoa in vitro. Fertil Steril 27:815–831, 1976.
81. Overstreet JW, Katz DF, Yudin AI: Cervical mucus and sperm transport in reproduction. Semin Perinatol 15:149–155, 1991.
82. Overstreet JW, Yanagimachi R, Katz DF, et al: Penetration of human spermatozoa into the human zona pellucida and zona-free hamster egg—a study of fertile donors and infertile patients. Fertil Steril 33:534–542, 1980.
83. Overstreet JW: Assessment of disorders of spermatogenesis. In Lockey JW, Lemasters GK, Keye WR (eds): Reproduction: The New Frontier in Occupational and Environmental Health Research. New York, Alan R. Liss, 1984, pp 275–292.
84. Overstreet JW: Semen liquefaction and viscosity problems. In Tanagho EA, Lue TF, McClure RD (eds): Contemporary Management of Impotence and Infertility. Baltimore, Willams & Wilkins, 1988, pp 311–312.
85. Overstreet JW: Evaluation of sperm-cervical mucus interaction. Fertil Steril 45:324–326, 1986.
86. Pandya IJ, Mortiner D, Sawers RS: A standardized approach for evaluating the penetration of human spermatozoa into cervical mucus in vitro. Fertil Steril 45:357–360, 1986.
87. Parslow JM, Poulton TA, Besser GM, et al: The clinical relevance of classes of immunoglobulins on spermatozoa from infertile and vasovasostomized males. Fertil Steril 43:621–627, 1985.
88. Patterson L, Jarow JP: Transrectal ultrasound in the evaluation of the infertile man. J Urol 144:1469–1471, 1990.
89. Pelfrey RJ, Overstreet JW, Lewis EL: Abnormalities of sperm morphology in cases of persistent infertility after vasectomy reversal. Fertil Steril 28:112–114, 1982.
90. Peng H-Q, Collins JA, Wilson EH, Wrixton W: Receiver-operating characteristics curves for semen analysis variables: Methods for evaluation of diagnostic tests of male gamete function. Gamete Res 17:229–236, 1987.
91. Polansky FF, Lamb EJ: Do the results of semen analysis predict future fertility? A survival analysis study. Fertil Steril 49:1059–1065, 1988.
92. Rehan NE, Sobrero AJ, Fertig JW: The semen of fertile men: Statistical analysis of 1300 men. Fertil Steril 26:492–502, 1975.
93. Rogers BJ: The sperm penetration assay: Its usefulness re-evaluated. Fertil Steril 43:821–840, 1985.
94. Rosen SW, Weintraub BD: Monotropic increase of serum FSH correlated with low sperm count in young men with oligospermia and aspermia. J Clin Endocrinol Metab 32:410–416, 1971.
95. Roth BJ, Williams SD: Complications of urologic chemotherapy. AUA Update Series 9:26, 1990.
96. Schrader SM: Occupational and environmental factors and male infertility. Infertil Reprod Med Clin North Am 3:319–328, 1992.
97. Sherins RJ, Howards SS: Male infertility. In Harrison JH, Gittes RF, Perlmutter AD, et al (eds): Campbell's Urology, Vol 1. Philadelphia, WB Saunders, 1978, p 715–776.
98. Silber SJ, Rodriquez-Rigau LI: Quantitative analysis of testicle biopsy: Determination of partial obstruction and prediction of sperm count after surgery for obstruction. Fertil Steril 36:480–485, 1981.
99. Singer R, Sagiv M, Barnet M, et al: Motility, vitality and percentages of morphologically abnormal forms of human spermatozoa in relation to sperm counts. Andrologia 12:92–96, 1980.
100. Smith DR: Critique on the concept of vesical neck obstruction in children. JAMA 207:1686–1692, 1969.
101. Sokol RZ: Medical and endocrine therapy of male factor infertility. Infertil Reprod Med Clin North Am 3:389–397, 1992.
102. Swartz D, Laplanche A, Jouannet P, David G: Within subject variabilities of human semen in regard to sperm count, volume, total number of spermatozoa and length of abstinence. J Reprod Fertil 57:391–395, 1979.
103. Swerdloff RS, Wang C, Sokol RZ: Endocrine evaluation of the infertile man. In Lipshultz LI, Howards SS (eds): Infertility in the Male. 2nd ed. St. Louis, Mosby, 1991, pp 211–222.
104. Tagatz GE, Okagai T, Sciarra JJ: The effect of vaginal lubricants on sperm motility and viability in vitro. Am J Obstet Gynecol 113:88–90, 1972.
105. Talbot P, Chacon RS: A new procedure for rapidly scoring acrosome reaction of human sperm. Gamete Res 3:211–216, 1980.
106. Tesarik J: Comparison of acrosome reaction-inducing activities of human cumulus oophorus, follicular fluid and ionophore A23187 in human sperm populations of proven fertilizing ability in vitro. J Reprod Fertil 74:383–388, 1985.

107. Turner TW, Schrader SM: Sperm morphometry as measured by three different computer systems. J Androl 9:P-45, 1988.
108. United States General Accounting Office: Reproductive and developmental toxicants. Washington, DC, US Govt Printing Office, 1991.
109. Van Thiel DH, Gavaler JS, Lester R, et al: Alcohol-induced testicular atrophy. Gastroenterology 69:326–332, 1975.
110. Van Thiel DH, Gavaler JS, Smith WI, et al: Hypothalamic-pituitary-gonadal dysfunction in men using cimetidine. N Engl J Med 300:1012–1015, 1979.
111. Van Thiel DH, Gavaler JS, Sanghvi A: Recovery of sexual function in abstinent alcoholic men. Gastroenterology 84:677–682, 1983.
112. Werner CA: Mumps orchitis and testicular atrophy. Ann Intern Med 32:1066–1074, 1950.
113. Wolf DP, Boldt J, Byrd W, Bechtol KB: Acrosomal status evaluation in human ejaculated sperm with monoclonal antibodies. Biol Reprod 32:1157–1162, 1985.
114. Wolff H, Anderson DJ: Immunohistologic characterization and quantitation of leukocyte subpopulations in human semen. Fertil Steril 49:497–504, 1988.
115. World Health Organization: WHO laboratory manual for the examination of human semen and sperm-cervical mucus interaction. 3rd ed. Cambridge, England, The Press Syndicate of the University of Cambridge, 1992.
116. World Health Organization: WHO manual for the examination of human semen and semen-cervical mucus interaction. 2nd ed. Cambridge, England, The Press Syndicate of the University of Cambridge, 1987.
117. Yanagimachi R, Lopata A, Odom CB, et al: Retention of biologic characteristics of zona pellucida in highly concentrated salt solution: The use of salt-stored eggs for assessing the fertilizing capacity of spermatozoa. Fertil Steril 31:562–574, 1979.
118. Yanagimachi R, Yanagimachi H, Rogers BJ: The use of zona-free animal ova as a system for the assessment of the fertilizing capacity of human spermatozoa. Biol Reprod 15:471–476, 1976.
119. Yanagimachi R: Mammalian fertilization. In Knobil E, Neill J (eds): The Physiology of Reproduction. Vol 1. New York, Raven, 1988, pp 135–175.
120. Yanagimachi R: Zona-free hamster eggs: Zona-free fertilizing capacity and examining chromosomes of human spermatozoa. Gamete Res 10:187–232, 1984.
121. Zamboni L: Sperm ultrastructural pathology as a cause of infertility. In Asch RH, Balmaceda JP, Johnston I (eds): Gamete Physiology. Norwell, MA, Serono Symposia, USA, 1990, pp 119–126.
122. Zanaveld LJD, Jeyendran RS: Modern assessment of semen for diagnostic purposes. Semin Reprod Endocrinol 6:324–337, 1988.
123. Zavos PM: Seminal parameters of ejaculates collected from oligospermic and normospermic patients via masturbation and at intercourse with the use of a Silastic seminal fluid collection device. Fertil Steril 44:517–520, 1985.
124. Zuckerman Z, Rodriquez-Rigau LJ, Smith KD, Steinberger E: Frequency distribution of sperm counts in fertile and infertile males. Fertil Steril 28:1310–1313, 1977.

STEVEN M. SCHRADER, PhD
M. HELEN KANITZ, PhD

OCCUPATIONAL HAZARDS TO MALE REPRODUCTION

From the Functional Toxicology
  Section (SMS)
  and
Experimental Toxicology Branch
  (MHK)
National Institute for Occupational
  Safety and Health
Robert A. Taft Laboratories
Cincinnati, Ohio

Reprint requests to:
Steven M. Schrader, PhD
Chief, Functional Toxicology
  Section
National Institute for Occupational
  Safety and Health
Robert A. Taft Laboratories
4676 Columbia Parkway
Mail Stop C23
Cincinnati, OH 45226

Research of the effects of toxicants on the male reproductive system in the occupational setting differ in the initiating factors, study design, and variables examined. The earliest report of occupational exposure dates back to 1775 when an English physician, Percivall Pott, reported a high incidence of scrotal cancer in chimney sweeps. This observation led to safety regulations in the form of bathing requirements for these workers.[63] While reproductive toxicology has been an area of interest during the intervening 200 years, the field was not firmly established until Lancranjan studied lead-exposed workers in Romania in 1975[31] and Whorton examined the effects of dibromochloropropane (DBCP) on male workers in California in 1977.[72] Since these discoveries, several additional human male reproductive toxicants have been identified by using clinical observations, population statistics, epidemiologic questionnaires, and hormonal and semen studies.

INITIATION OF STUDIES

Many factors influence the decision to study a group of workers. Studies of DBCP were initiated after informal discussions of infertility problems among wives attending a softball game.[71] A physician noting a cluster of infertile patients from a specific occupation (e.g., the professional truck driver[55]) may initiate a study. The petroleum refinery industry exemplifies a profession in which the workers themselves had concerns regarding their reproductive health.[52] Work-related accidents, such as the chemical spill of bromide[49] or the nuclear radiation disaster in Chernobyl,[3] also have led to studies. Corporations may conduct occupational research to validate previous claims as with studies on dinitrotoluene (DNT) and toluene diamine (TDA).[23] In Europe, epidemiologic comparisons of fertility and paternal occupation have been readily made, since parents' work records are linked to birth records in these countries. The majority of epidemiologic and occupational research, however, has been stimulated by data from animal studies indicating that a compound is a reproductive toxicant. Thus, the toxicologist, the physician, the epidemiologist, the worker himself, the labor union, and the corporation have been and will continue to be "on the lookout" for potential exposures and study populations.

These alerts have triggered several different approaches to defining the nature and extent of the effect. Some of these study designs are described below.

POPULATION-BASED STUDIES

Population-based studies (Table 1) link job title and/or description with reproductive outcome. Because adverse pregnancies are generally rare events, large populations must be studied to detect most significant associations. Although in some areas of the United States medical birth records do not reveal parental occupation, this type of study is routinely conducted in European countries, where the parents' work history is included in medical records. These record-based population studies are problematic, however, in that they preclude control for potentially confounding lifestyle factors such as alcohol consumption and drug abuse.

TABLE 1. Population-based Studies of Paternal Effects

Reference	Type of Exposure or Occupation	Association with Exposure	Effect
Lindbohm et al.[39]	Solvents	−	Spontaneous abortion
Lindbohm et al.[39]	Service station	+	Spontaneous abortion
Daniell and Vaughan[12]	Organic solvents	−	Spontaneous abortion
McDonald et al.[41]	Mechanics	+	Spontaneous abortion
McDonald et al.[41]	Food processing	+	Developmental defects
Lindbohm et al.[38]	Ethylene oxide	+	Spontaneous abortion
Lindbohm et al.[38]	Petroleum refinery	+	Spontaneous abortion
Lindbohm et al.[38]	Impregnants of wood	+	Spontaneous abortion
Lindbohm et al.[38]	Rubber chemicals	+	Spontaneous abortion
Olsen et al.[48]	Metals	+	Child cancer risk
Olsen et al.[48]	Machinists	+	Child cancer risk
Olsen et al.[48]	Smiths	+	Child cancer risk
Kristensen et al.[29]	Solvents	+	Preterm birth
Kristensen et al.[29]	Lead and solvents	+	Preterm birth
Kristensen et al.[29]	Lead	+	Perinatal death
Kristensen et al.[29]	Lead	+	Male child morbidity

− no significant association
+ significant association
Adapted from Taskinen H: Effects of parental occupational exposures on spontaneous abortion and congenital malformation. Scand J Work Environ Health 16:297–314, 1990.

Another major problem with population-based studies is the possibility of nondifferential misclassification of exposure. For example, pesticide exposure of such heterogeneous professions as crop farming and fishery husbandry may be very different even though these two groups are often classified together. Differentiation of exposure is difficult even if the International Standard Industrial Classification system is used. For example Code 92012, Refuse Removal Activities, combines cleaning companies, dumps, and incinerators, but employees of cleaning companies are not subjected to the levels of ash and pyrolysis products to which incinerator operators are commonly exposed. This drawback may make it more difficult to correctly identify a toxic effect on reproduction.

Population-based studies have caused a new surge of interest in male-mediated adverse pregnancy outcomes.[10] Several reports (*see* Table 1) have shown that paternal exposure may affect pregnancy or the health of the offspring. These data have stimulated research into the genetic stability of the sperm cell and the cause/effect relationships of damage to sperm.[13]

CASE-CONTROL STUDIES

Case-control or case-referent studies (Table 2) involve comparing the frequency of toxic exposure of persons who have experienced reproductive dysfunction to those without such a medical history.[35] The exposure history of

TABLE 2. Case-control Studies of Paternal Effects

Reference	Type of Exposure or Occupation	Association with Exposure	Effect
Kucera[30]	Printing industry	(+)	Cleft lip
Kucera[30]	Paint	(+)	Cleft palate
Olsen[47]	Paint	+	Damage to central nervous system
Olsen[47]	Solvents	(+)	Damage to central nervous system
Sever et al.[62]	Low level radiation	+	Neural tube defects
Taskinen et al.[65]	Organic solvents	+	Spontaneous abortion
Taskinen et al.[65]	Aromatic hydrocarbons	+	Spontaneous abortion
Taskinen et al.[65]	Dust	+	Spontaneous abortion
Gardner et al.[19]	Radiation	+	Childhood leukemia
Bonde[7]	Welding	+	Time to conception
Wilkins and Sinks[75]	Agriculture	(+)	Child brain tumor
Wilkins and Sinks[75]	Construction	(+)	Child brain tumor
Wilkins and Sinks[75]	Food/tobacco processing	(+)	Child brain tumor
Wilkins and Sinks[75]	Metal	+	Child brain tumor
Lindbohm et al.[40]	Lead	(+)	Spontaneous abortion
Sallmen et al.[53]	Lead	(+)	Congenital defects
Veulemans et al.[66]	Ethylene glycol ether	+	Abnormal spermiogram
Chia et al.[8]	Metals	+	Cadmium in semen

(+) marginally significant association
 + significant association
Adapted from Taskinen H: Effects of parental occupational exposures on spontaneous abortion and congenital malformation. Scand J Work Environ Health 16:297–314, 1990.

each group is determined by interviews and other data sources. Like population-based studies, case-control studies provide an efficient design to detect the association of rare outcomes with toxic exposures. However, in this type of study, recall bias may yield misleading results. A person who has experienced an adverse outcome may report an exposure more readily than one with no history of reproductive dysfunction. As Levin describes,[35] a couple that has recently experienced a stillbirth or had a congenitally malformed child may be more inclined to search for a previous toxic exposure as the source. Another potential source of bias in these studies exists with the interviewer, who should be "blind" to the reproductive status and the exposure classification of the respondent.

STANDARDIZED FERTILITY RATIO

The standardized fertility or birth ratio (SFR) (Table 3) compares the number of observed births within a population to the number of expected births. The latter value is obtained using the birth rate of an external population. To monitor a specific workforce group, Wong[76] uses a simple standardization method to provide noninvasive, readily available data. His method uses a couple's reproductive history to measure male fecundity. The number of expected births is obtained from the birth rate for U.S. women of the same age group. There are some problems with this simplified approach. Since the U.S. birth rate, as collected by the National Center for Health Statistics, does not take into account marital status, birth control for frequency of intercourse,[37] there is the potential for a positive or negative bias in making such comparisons. Wong's method erroneously assumes all women to be equally libidinous and fecund. Additionally, since only married men are evaluated in SFR studies, there are age-related restrictions in the data as well as a likely underestimate of the number of children born out of wedlock. Some researchers have tried to correct for these variations using different models.[36,37] It appears that the SFR overestimates the birth rate in both control and exposed populations, even when a reduction in semen quality exists.[68] Levine[36] suggests the SFR would be a reliable indicator in a cohort study in which both the control and comparison populations are selected on the same basis.

COHORT STUDIES

Cohort studies (Table 4) evaluate the frequency of adverse reproductive outcome between exposed and unexposed groups. Cross-sectional cohort studies

TABLE 3. Standardized Birth Ratio Studies of Male Fertility Effects

Reference	Type of Exposure or Occupation	Association with Exposure
Wong et al.[76]	Ethylene dibromide	(+)
Levine[37]	DBCP	+
Hamill et al.[23]	TDA and DNT	−
Lauwerys et al.[32]	Mercury	−
Lauwerys et al.[32]	Manganese	+
Welch et al.[68]	Ethylene glycol ether	−
Lemasters et al.[33]	Chemical contaminated sewage	−

− no significant association
(+) marginally significant association
 + significant association

TABLE 4. Cohort Studies of Male Reproductive Effects

Reference	Type of Study	Type of Exposure	Effect
Lancranjan et al.[31]	Questionnaire, semen	Lead	Semen quality, sexual function
Whorton et al.[73]	Questionnaire, semen, endocrine	DBCP	Semen quality, endocrine function
Whorton et al.[74]	Questionnaire, semen, endocrine	Carbaryl (Sevin)	None
Milby and Whorton[44]	Questionnaire, semen	DBCP	Semen quality
Milby and Whorton[44]	Questionnaire, semen	Epichlorohyrdrin	None
Wyrobek et al.[77]	Questionnaire, semen	Carbaryl (Sevin)	Semen quality
Meyer[43]	Questionniare, semen	carbon disulfide	
Ahrenholtz and Meyer[1]	Questionnaire, semen	TDA and DNT	Semen quality
Hamill et al.[23]	Questionnaire, semen, endocrine	TDA and DNT	None
Nordstrom et al.[46]	Questionnaire, records	High voltage	Congenital malformations
Ward et al.[67]	Questionnaire, semen	Formaldehyde	None
Goldsmith and Potashnik[22]	Questionnaire	DBCP	Sex ratio in offspring (favors females)
Rosenburg et al.[52]	Semen	Petroleum refinery	None
Heussner et al.[24]	Questionnaire, semen	Coal tar pitch	None
Assemmato et al.[2]	Questionnaire, semen, endocrine	Lead	Semen quality, not endocrine
Ratcliffe et al.[51]	Questionnaire, semen	Ethylene dibromide	Semen quality
Schrader et al.[61]	Questionnaire, semen	Ethylene dibromide	Semen quality
Jelnes[26]	Questionnaire, semen, endocrine	Styrene and acetone (plastic production)	Semen quality
Jelnes and Knudsen[27]	Semen	Stainless steel weld	None
Welch et al.[69]	Questionnaire, semen, endocrine	Ethylene glycol ethers	Semen quality
Ratcliffe et al.[50]	Questionnaire, semen	Ethylene glycol ethers	Semen quality
DeStefano et al.[14]	Questionnaire, semen, endocrine	Military—Vietnam	Semen quality
Bonde[4]	Semen	Welding	Semen effects not reversible
Bonde[5]	Semen, endocrine	Welding	Semen quality
Bonde et al.[6]	Questionnaire, birth records	Welding	Fertility (mild steel)
Eskenazi et al.[16]	Semen	Perchloroethylene	Semen quality
Eskenazi et al.[15]	Questionnaire	Perchloroethylene	Time to pregnancy
Ng et al.[45]	Endocrine	Lead	Endocrine function
McGregor and Mason[42]	Questionnaire, endocrine	Mercury vapor	Sex hormone binding globulin
Figa-Talamanca et al.[17]	Questionnaire, semen	Heat	Semen quality and conception
Weyandt et al.[70]	Questionnaire, semen, endocrine	Radar	Semen quality
Gennart et al.[20]	Questionnaire, endocrine	Lead	None
Gennart et al.[21]	Questionnaire	Lead	Fertility
Hoglund et al.[25]	Questionnaire	Spray paint	Birth weight and length
Lerda[34]	Semen	Lead	Semen quality

evaluate the groups as they currently exist, whereas historical cohort studies are conducted on previously exposed and unexposed groups. An example of the latter is the 1989 Vietnam experience study, in which military veterans were grouped according to whether they had served in Vietnam from 1967–1972.[14] This study was able to detect subsequent differences between the groups in semen quality and time to pregnancy but revealed little about the reproductive health of the individuals at the time of exposure.

A cohort study may be longitudinal (prospective). In such a study, baseline data are collected, and individuals are studied over time for a specific reproductive outcome. A longitudinal study is exemplified by the study of "summer hire" pesticide applicators.[61] Individuals were evaluated at the beginning of the season before they started working with pesticides and at the conclusion of the spraying season two months later. This study illustrates the importance of selecting appropriate variables for a study design. If semen analyses are conducted to predict reproductive outcome, the correct timing is needed. Since the time for spermatogenesis and delivery of mature sperm to the ejaculate is approximately 72 days, if primary spermatogonia were affected by exposure, this would not be observed in a time frame that covered less than 80–90 days. Thus, the study of "summer hire" workers could not make valid conclusions regarding the effect on spermatogenesis of a 2-month exposure among pesticide applicators.

Cohort studies may involve questionnaires, neuroendocrine measurements, semen analyses, or a combination of these. Questionnaire studies are advantageous in that they are the least expensive and least invasive. As with case-control studies, however, inherent problems exist such as possible interviewer bias and the potential for selective memory of respondents (particularly in a historical cohort study) who have experienced an adverse outcome. Additionally, many cohort studies lack an adequate number of pregnancies needed to detect differences between groups.[60]

Studies evaluating the neuroendocrine system measure male hormones in blood samples. Although blood sampling is a widely accepted medical practice, it is an invasive procedure, and the endocrine profile does not necessarily reflect the status of the male reproductive system.[2] Semen analysis provides information on spermatogenesis, accessory sex glands, and sperm cell motility.[59] Studies using semen samples require the participants to produce samples by masturbation, and there are concerns regarding participation bias.[37] Additionally, this procedure employs complex scientific equipment and methodologies.[58] Cohort studies that combine all the above approaches provide the most information and thus the greatest likelihood of detecting adverse reproductive effects. However, such studies are expensive, complex, and necessitate a team approach minimally requiring an (1) andrologist, (2) epidemiologist, (3) industrial hygienist, (4) physician, and (5) statistician.[57]

CLINICAL STUDIES

Clinical or case studies (Table 5) involve the report by a physician of workers exposed to potentially toxic agents. These reports involve the evaluation of individuals, groups of workers of the same occupation or exposure, or clinical treatment following accidental exposure. While such reports rarely provide a definitive relationship between exposure and male reproductive effects, they can serve as sentinel reports that initiate further studies.

Some clinical studies provide unique information that would not be observed by using other methods. A clinical study of a firearms instructor[18] provided

TABLE 5. Clinical/Case Studies of Male Reproductive Effects

Reference	Type of Study	Type of Exposure	Association with Exposure	Effect
Whorton et al.[72]	Cluster	DBCP	+	Semen quality, endocrine function
Cohn et al.[9]	Case report	Kepone	+	Semen quality
Cullen et al.[11]	Medical monitor	Lead	+	Semen quality
Kelly[28]	Case report	Methylene chloride	+	Semen quality
Fisher-Fischbein et al.[18]	Case report	Lead	+	Semen quality
Potashnik et al.[49]	Accident	Bromine vapor	+	Semen quality
Birioukov et al.[3]	Accident	Radiation	+	Semen quality, endocrine function

+ significant association

possibly the best demonstration of the effect of lead on sperm. The instructor had fathered one son but became infertile as a result of work exposure that elevated his blood lead concentration to 88 μg/dL. During the next 3 years the exposure was decreased, and the man was placed on chelation therapy. His sperm count increased as his blood levels decreased, and he subsequently fathered another child after his blood level of lead decreased below 30 μg/dL. Similarly, after men exposed to high levels of kepone in the work environment were treated with cholestyramine to offset the toxic action of kepone, their sperm count and sperm motility increased accordingly.[9]

Work-related accidents may provide case study data on high-level exposures. These in turn may indicate the parameters to be studied at lower exposures.

SURVEILLANCE OF MALE REPRODUCTION

A surveillance strategy for evaluating men working with known male reproductive toxicants was proposed and conducted by a team from the University of California.[56] However, this program had many problems and was eventually discontinued.[54] While this first attempt was discouraging, chemicals such as lead and ethylene glycol ethers remain in the U.S. workplace, posing a hazard to the reproductive health of the male worker. A surveillance program is needed to monitor those working with these and other occupational toxicants.

In the future, strong reproductive data is needed not only to identify the scope of the problem but also to protect the health of these men and their potential offspring.

REFERENCES

1. Ahrenholz SH, Meyer CR: Health hazard evaluation determination report: Olin Chemical Company. Cincinnati, NIOSH, 1980, US Dept of Health and Human Services publication HHE 79-113-728.
2. Assennato G, Paci C, Baser ME, et al: Sperm count suppression without endocrine dysfunction in lead-exposed men. Arch Environ Health 41:387–390, 1986.
3. Birioukov A, Meurer M, Peter RU, et al: Male reproductive system in patients exposed to ionizing irradiation in the Chernobyl accident. Arch Androl 3:99–104, 1993.
4. Bonde JP: Semen quality in welders before and after three weeks of non-exposure. Br J Ind Med 47:515–518, 1990.
5. Bonde JP: Semen quality and sex hormones among mild steel and stainless steel welders—a cross sectional study. Br J Ind Med 47:508–514, 1990.

6. Bonde JP, Hansen KS, Levine RJ: Fertility among Danish male welders. Scand J Work Environ Health 16:315–322, 1990.

7. Bonde JPE: Subfertility in relation to welding—a case referent study among male welders. Dan Med Bull 37:105–108, 1990.

8. Chia SE, Ong CN, Lee ST, Tsakok FHM: Blood concentration of lead, cadmium, mercury, zinc, and copper and human semen parameters. Arch Androl 29:177–183, 1992.

9. Cohn WJ, Boylan JJ, Blanke RV, et al: Treatment of chlordecone (kepone) toxicity with cholestyramine; results of a controlled clinical trial. N Engl J Med 298:243–248, 1978.

10. Colie CF: Male mediated teratogenesis. Reprod Toxicol 7:3–9, 1993.

11. Cullen MR, Kaye RD, Robins JM: Endocrine and reproductive dysfunction in men associated with occupational inorganic lead intoxication. Arch Environ Health 39:431–440, 1984.

12. Daniell WE, Vaughan TL: Paternal employment in solvent related occupations and adverse pregnancy outcomes. Br J Ind Med 45:193–197, 1988.

13. Davis DL, Friedler G, Mattison D, Morris R: Male medicated teratogenesis and other reproductive effects—biologic and epidemiologic findings and a plea for clinical research. Reprod Toxicol 6:289–292, 1992.

14. Destefano F, Annest JL, Kresnow MJ, et al: Semen characteristics of Vietnam veterans. Reprod Toxicol 3:165–173, 1989.

15. Eskenazi BE, Fenster L, Hudes M, et al: A study of the effect of perchloroethylene exposure on the reproductive outcomes of wives of dry cleaning workers. Am J Ind Med 20:593–600, 1991.

16. Eskenazi BE, Wyrobek AJ, Fenster L, et al: A study of the effect of perchloroethylene exposure on semen quality in dry cleaning workers. Am J Ind Med 20:575–591, 1991.

17. Figa-Talamamca I, Dell'Orco V, Pupi A, et al: Fertility and semen quality of workers exposed to high temperature in the ceramics industry. Reprod Toxicol 6:517–523, 1992.

18. Fisher-Fischbein J, Fischbein A, Melnick HD, Bardin CW: Correlation between biochemical indicators of lead exposure and semen quality in a lead-poisoned firearms instructor. JAMA 257:803–805, 1987.

19. Gardner MJ, Hall AJ, Snee MP, et al: Methods and basic design of case-control study of leukemia and lymphoma among young people near Sellafield nuclear plant in West Cumbria. Br Med J 300:429–434, 1990.

20. Gennart JP, Bernard A, Lauwerys R: Assessment of thyroid, testes, kidney and autonomic nervous system function in lead-exposed workers. Int Arch Occup Environ Health 64:49–57, 1992.

21. Gennart JP, Buchet JP, Roels H, et al: Fertility of male workers exposed to cadmium, lead, or manganese. Am J Epidemiol 135:1209–1219, 1992.

22. Goldsmith JR, Potashnik G: Reproductive outcomes in families of DBCP-exposed men. Arch Environ Med 39:85–89, 1984.

23. Hamill PVV, Steinberger E, Levine RJ, et al: The epidemiologic assessment of male reproductive hazard from occupational exposure to TDA and DNT. J Occup Med 24:985–993, 1982.

24. Heussner JC, Ward JB, Legator MS: Genetic monitoring of aluminum workers exposed to coal tar pitch volatiles. Mutat Res 155:143–155, 1985.

25. Hoglund GV, Iselius EL, Knave BG: Children of male spray painters-weight and length at birth. Br J Ind Med 49:249–253, 1992.

26. Jelnes JE: Semen quality in workers producing reinforced plastic. Reprod Toxicol 2:209–212, 1988.

27. Jelnes JE, Knudson LE: Stainless steel welding and semen quality. Reprod Toxicol 2:213–215, 1988.

28. Kelly M: Case reports of individuals with oligospermia and methylene chloride exposures. Reprod Toxicol 2:13–17, 1988.

29. Kristensen P, Irgens LM, Daltveit AK, Andersen A: Perinatal outcome among children of men exposed to lead and organic solvents in the printing industry. Am J Epidemiol 137:134–144, 1993.

30. Kucera J: Exposure to fat solvents: A possible cause of sacral agenesis in man. J Pediatr 72:857–859, 1968.

31. Lancranjan I, Popescu HI, Gavanescu O, et al: Reproductive ability of workmen occupationally exposed to lead. Arch Environ Health 30:396–401, 1975.

32. Lauwerys, Roels RH, Genet P, et al: Fertility of male workers exposed to mercury vapor or to manganese dust: A questionnaire study. Am J Ind Med 7:171–176, 1985.

33. Lemasters GK, Zenick H, Hertzberg V, Hansen K, Clark S: Fertility of workers chronically exposed to chemically contaminated sewer wastes. Reprod Toxicol 5:31–37, 1991.

34. Lerda D: Study of sperm characteristics in persons occupationally exposed to lead. Am J Ind Med 22:567–571, 1992.

35. Levin SM: Problems and pitfalls in conducting epidemiological research in the area of reproductive toxicology. Am J Ind Med 4:349–364, 1983.
36. Levine RJ: Monitoring fertility to detect toxicity to the male reproductive system. Reprod Toxicol 2:223–227, 1988.
37. Levine RJ, Blunden PB, Dalcorso D, et al: Superiority of reproductive histories to sperm count in detecting infertility at dibromochloropropane manufacturing plant. J Occup Med 25:591–597, 1983.
38. Lindbohm M-L, Hemminki K, Bonhomme MG, et al: Effects of paternal occupational exposure on spontaneous abortions. Am J Pub Health 81:1029–1033, 1991.
39. Lindbohm M-L, Hemminki K, Kyyronen P: Parental occupational exposure and spontaneous abortions in Finland. Am J Epidemiol 120:370–378, 1984.
40. Lindbohm M-L, Sallmen M, Anttila A, et al: Paternal occupational lead exposure and spontaneous abortion. Scand J Work Environ Health 17:95–103, 1991.
41. McDonald AD, McDonald JC, Armstrong B, et al: Fathers' occupation and pregnancy outcome. Br J Ind Med 46:329–333, 1989.
42. McGregor AJ, Mason HJ: Occupational mercury vapour exposure and testicular, pituitary and thyroid endocrine function. Hum Exper Toxicol 10:199–203, 1991.
43. Meyer CR: Semen quality in workers exposed to carbon disulfide compared to a control group from the same plant. J Occup Med 323:435–439, 1981.
44. Milby TH, Worton D: Epidemiological assessment of occupationally related chemically induced sperm count suppression. J Occup Med 22:77–82, 1980.
45. Ng TP, Goh HH, Ng YL, et al: Male endocrine functions in workers with moderate exposure to lead. Br J Ind Med 48:485–491, 1991.
46. Nordstrom S, Birke E, Gustavsson L: Reproductive hazards among workers at high voltage substations. Bioelectromagnetics 4:91–101, 1983.
47. Olsen J: Risk of exposure to teratogens amongst laboratory staff and painters. Dan Med Bull 30:24–28, 1983.
48. Olsen JH, Brown PDN, Schulgen G, Jensen OM: Parental employment at time of conception and risk of cancer in offspring. Eur J Cancer 27:958–965, 1991.
49. Potashnik G, Carel R, Belmaker I, Levine M: Spermatogenesis and reproductive performance following human accidental exposure to bromine vapor. Reprod Toxicol 6:171–174, 1992.
50. Ratcliffe JM, Schrader SM, Clapp DE, et al: Semen quality in workers exposed to 2-ethoxyethanol. Br J Ind Med 46:399–406, 1989.
51. Ratcliffe JM, Schrader SM, Steenland K, et al: Semen quality in papaya workers with long term exposure to ethylene dibromide. Br J Ind Med 44:317–326, 1987.
52. Rosenberg MJ, Wyrobek AJ, Ratcliffe J, et al: Sperm as an indicator of reproductive risk among petroleum refinery workers. Br J Ind Med 42:123–127, 1985.
53. Sallmen M, Lindbohm ML, Anttila A, et al: Paternal occupational lead exposure and congenital malformations. J Epidemiol Community Health 46:519–522, 1992.
54. Samuels SJ: Lessons from a surveillance program of semen quality. Reprod Toxicol 2:229–231, 1988.
55. Sas M, Szollosi J: Impaired spermatogenesis as a common finding among professional drivers. Arch Androl 3:57–60, 1979.
56. Schenker MB, Samuels SJ, Perkins C, et al: Prospective surveillance of semen quality in the workplace. J Occup Med 30:336–344, 1988.
57. Schrader SM: General techniques for assessing male reproductive potential in human field studies. In Chapin R, Heindel J (eds): Methods in Reproductive Toxicology. Vol 3A. San Diego, 1993, pp 362–371.
58. Schrader SM, Chapin RE, Clegg ED, et al: Laboratory methods for assessing human semen in epidemiologic studies: A consensus report. Reprod Toxicol 6:275–279, 1992.
59. Schrader SM, Kesner JS: Mechanisms of male reproductive toxicology. In Paul M (ed): Occupational and Environmental Reproductive Hazards: A Guide for Clinicians. Baltimore, Williams & Wilkins, 1992, pp 3–17.
60. Schrader SM, Ratcliffe JM, Turner TW, Hornung RW: The use of new field methods of semen analysis in the study of occupational hazards to reproduction: The example of ethylene dibromide. J Occup Med 29:963–966, 1987.
61. Schrader SM, Turner TW, Ratcliffe JM: The effects of ethylene dibromide on semen quality: A comparison of short term and chronic exposure. Reprod Toxicol 2:191–198, 1988.
62. Sever LE, Gilbert ES, Hessol NA, McIntyre JM: A case-control study of congenital malformations and occupational exposure to low-level radiation. Am J Epidemiol 127:226–242, 1988.
63. Sherman IW, Sherman VG: Biology: A Human Approach. New York, Oxford University Press, 1979, pp 153–154.

64. Taskinen H: Effects of parental occupational exposures on spontaneous abortion and congenital malformation. Scand J Work Environ Health 16:297–314, 1990.
65. Taskinen H, Anttila A, Lindbohm ML, et al: Spontaneous abortions and congenital malformations among the wives of men occupationally exposed to organic solvents. Scand J Work Environ Health 15:345–352, 1989.
66. Veulemans H, Steeno O, Masschelein R, Groesneken D: Exposure to ethylene glycol ethers and spermatogenic disorders in man: A case-control study. Br J Ind Med 50:71–78, 1993.
67. Ward JB, Hokanson JA, Smith ER, et al: Sperm count, morphology and fluorescent body frequency in autopsy service workers exposed to formaldehyde. Mutat Res 130:417–424, 1984.
68. Welch LS, Plotkin E, Schrader S: Indirect fertility analysis in painters exposed to ethylene glycol ethers: Sensitivity and specificity. Am J Ind Med 20:229–240, 1991.
69. Welch LS, Schrader SM, Turner TW, Cullen MR: Effects of exposure to ethylene glycol ethers on shipyard painters: II. Male reproduction. Am J Ind Med 14:509–526, 1988.
70. Weyandt TB, Schrader SM, Turner TW, Simon SD: Semen analysis of military personnel associated with military duty assignments. J Androl 13:29, 1992.
71. Whorton D, Foliart D: DBCP: Eleven years later. Presented at the Symposium on the Assessment of Reproductive Hazards in the Workplace. Cincinnati, June 16, 1988.
72. Whorton D, Krauss RM, Marshall S, Milby TH: Infertility in male pesticide workers. Lancet 2:1259–1260, 1977.
73. Whorton MD, Milby TH, Krauss RM, Stubbs HA: Testicular function in DBCP exposed pesticide workers. J Occup Med 21:161–166, 1979.
74. Whorton MD, Milby TH, Stubbs HA, et al: Testicular function among carbaryl-exposed employees. J Toxicol Environ Health 5:929–941, 1979.
75. Wilkins JR, Sinks T: Parental occupation and intracranial neoplasms of childhood: Results of a case-control interview study. Am J Epidemiol 132:275–292, 1990.
76. Wong O, Utidijian HMD, Karten VS: Retrospective evaluation of reproductive performance of workers exposed to ethylene dibromide (EDB). J Occup Med 21:98–102, 1979.
77. Wyrobek AJ, Watchmaker G, Gordon L, et al: Sperm shape abnormalities in carbaryl-exposed employees. Environ Health Perspec 40:225–265, 1981.

ANTHONY P. CHEUNG, MB BS, MPH,
FRACOG, FRCS(C)

CLINICAL APPROACH TO FEMALE REPRODUCTIVE PROBLEMS

From the Department of Obstetrics
  and Gynaecology
University of Alberta
Edmonton, Alberta
Canada

Reprint requests to:
Anthony P. Cheung
Assistant Professor
Department of Obstetrics and
  Gynaecology
1D1 Mackenzie Health Sciences
  Centre
University of Alberta
Edmonton, Alberta
Canada T6G 2R7

The possible association of occupational hazards and female reproduction is summarized in other chapters. The focus of this chapter is to outline the clinician's approach to female reproductive problems. To follow the themes in other chapters in this review, this chapter will focus on the clinical approach to the management of infertility with a brief outline of the management of recurrent abortion and antenatal diagnosis. The discussion of ovarian dysfunction will be in relation to infertility only rather than a comprehensive review of the subject.

INFERTILITY

The fecundability, or monthly probability of conception, in a normal population has been estimated to be approximately 20%.[5] Infertility is defined as an inability to conceive after 12 months of trying. The etiologic factors include male reproductive dysfunction, ovulatory dysfunction, tubal/pelvic factors, and uterine and cervical factors. In some instances, infertility has been attributed to an immunological cause. Finally, there remains a subset of infertile couples in which no abnormalities can be identified after thorough investigation. These couples are considered to have "unexplained" infertility. The clinical approach to male reproductive problems is discussed in detail in chapter 3 and will not be repeated here.

Ovulatory Dysfunction

A careful menstrual history frequently can indicate the ovulatory status of a woman of reproductive age. Regular monthly menses associated with cyclical premenstrual molimina (breast tenderness, abdominal bloating, fluid retention, mood change) and menstrual cramps are suggestive of an ovulatory cycle. These symptoms, however, occur in various frequency and degree among different individuals. A recent increase in the severity of menstrual cramps may suggest other symptoms that may provide a clue to a potential cause of infertility such as uterine fibroids or endometriosis. It is important, though, to emphasize that these are only "soft" symptoms and may have no significance in isolation. Some women also experience a midcycle increase in cervical mucus. This is related to the marked increase in circulating estradiol levels for 2–3 days prior to ovulation. Under the influence of estradiol, cervical mucus increases in amount, becomes watery and stretchy (spinnbarkeit) and, when spread out and dried on a glass slide, forms the typical "ferning" pattern observed under light microscopy. These features are used to various degree in the Billings' method of contraception and the postcoital test as part of the infertility work-up. Ovulatory dysfunction typically manifests as oligo-ovulation or chronic anovulation. From the clinical standpoint, it is divided into those with normal estrogen effect and those with low estrogen effect.

Normal Estrogen

Normal estrogen is easily distinguished by the progestogen challenge test. Endometrium proliferates under the stimulation of endogenous estrogen in the normal follicular phase. Following ovulation, progesterone dominates and converts the endometrium to a secretory pattern. In the absence of pregnancy, the corpus luteum undergoes degeneration. This is accompanied by a fall in circulating estrogen and progesterone levels and the onset of menses. In anovulation associated with normal early- to midfollicular phase levels of estrogen, endometrial shedding, or "progestogen withdrawal bleeding," can be induced following the administration of progestogen (e.g., Provera, 10 mg daily) for 7–10 days. If endogenous estrogen levels are low, progestogen withdrawal bleeding will be absent. In women with normal endogenous estrogen levels, two subgroups of anovulation can be conveniently distinguished by the presence or absence of hyperandrogenism.

No Hyperandrogenism.   Patients with anovulation but no evidence of hyperandrogenism are normal otherwise and usually have weight appropriate for their height. Occasionally, compensated hypothyroid disease and mild hyperprolactinemia may be an underlying cause. Therefore, in these patients, prior to inducing ovulation, a serum thyroid-stimulating hormone (TSH) and prolactin level should be evaluated. Clomiphene citrate (Clomid or Serophene) is the treatment of choice. These women, in general, respond very well to clomiphene citrate in terms of successful ovulation and pregnancy once the optimal dose is identified.

A special group in this category is Asherman's syndrome, in which ovulatory function is in fact normal, but there is decreased or absent menstrual flow. Diagnosis is suggested by the characteristic menstrual history. Typically, secondary amenorrhea or hypomenorrhea develops following a recent dilatation and curettage (D&C). Despite the lack of menses, cyclical premenstrual molimina and menstrual-like cramping are present. This is due to intrauterine adhesions or synechiae and, in some instances, in combination with cervical stenosis. It is thought that an important precipitating factor is a vigorous D&C performed at a time when the uterus is most vulnerable, as in the puerperium. Investigation includes hysterosalpingography (HSG) and hysteroscopy. An HSG will show the uterine synechiae as filling defects with sharp, serpiginous margins and can show the extent of uterine cavity involved. Hysteroscopy further defines the nature of the adhesions (dense versus filmy; avascular versus vascular) and allows therapeutic dissection and separation at the same time. Postoperatively, a brief period of estrogen replacement is frequently introduced to help rejuvenate the endometrium.

Evidence of Hyperandrogenism. Patients with hyperandrogenism are commonly diagnosed as having polycystic ovarian syndrome (PCOS).[3] Hyperandrogenism is a hallmark in this condition, and the orderly hormonal changes in the normal cycle dynamics are absent. In the case of marked hirsutism and/or evidence of virilism, investigation includes measurement of serum testosterone (T), and dehydroepiandrosterone sulphate (DHEAS) levels. T and DHEAS serve as markers for a potential androgen-secreting ovarian tumor and adrenal tumor, respectively. A cutoff level of 200 ng/dL ($\approx$ 7 nmol/L) for T and 700 μg/dL (19 μmol/L) for DHEAS has been used to decide if further investigation should be initiated to exclude an ovarian tumor (pelvic ultrasound) or an adrenal tumor (CT scan). If the patient's mother and/or female siblings also have chronic anovulation and hirsutism, adult-onset congenital adrenal hyperplasia (CAH), which can mimic PCOS, should be excluded. Since 21-hydroxylase deficiency is the most common cause of CAH, a serum 17-hydroxyprogesterone level is used to screen for this condition. If the level is more than 300 ng/dL (9 nmol/L), further testing with an ACTH stimulation test will be necessary.[10] Obesity is a common feature of PCOS, and in some circumstances it may be difficult to distinguish PCOS from Cushing's syndrome. A dexamethasone suppression test may be necessary to differentiate the two conditions. The first choice of treatment to induce ovulation is clomiphene citrate. If DHEAS is mildly elevated but not in the range when an adrenal tumor is suspected, the judicious administration of a corticosteroid to suppress the elevated adrenal androgen levels encountered in these women with PCOS may improve their ovulatory rates to clomiphene citrate. However, a subset of women with PCOS remains unresponsive to clomiphene citrate and eventually requires the use of gonadotropins. Various regimens using follicle-stimulating hormone, or combinations of FSH and leutinizing hormone (LH) with or without prior gonadotropin-releasing hormone (GnRH) agonist suppression have been used. Because these patients can be very sensitive to gonadotropin treatment, careful monitoring of ovarian response with serial serum estradiol levels and pelvic ultrasound is essential. Recently, laparoscopic cautery of the multiple follicles present in the polycystic ovaries has been introduced as an alternative. However, if these women fail to get pregnant following this surgical treatment, anovulation commonly returns. Potentially, periovarian adhesions may develop following this approach.

LOW ESTROGEN

Normal or Low Serum FSH. Patients with low estrogen invariably present with amenorrhea. Manifestations of low endogenous estrogen are similar to those encountered in menopause. Symptoms include hot flushes, dry vagina, and, hence, dyspareunia. Physical examination may demonstrate decreased breast size and little or absent cervical mucus. Some hypothalamic causes are severe weight loss, emotional stress, and excessive exercise such as by marathon runners. Normalization of these factors may help to reestablish normal menstrual function or improve the response to ovulation induction with hormones. Rarely, a hypothalamic lesion is an underlying cause. A relatively common pituitary cause is a prolactin-secreting microadenoma. In the initial phase, these patients may present with normal ovulatory function or oligo-ovulation with or without galactorrhea and have normal estrogen levels with respect to end-organ response. In more florid cases, amenorrhea associated with low estrogen with or without galactorrhea predominates. A serum prolactin level is an important screening test. If it is significantly elevated and is not related to stress, drugs, or thyroid disease, further testing to exclude a pituitary prolactin-secreting tumor is paramount. While it has been suggested that a skull x-ray (cone-view) will serve as a screening test for a pituitary tumor, it remains less than optimal with respect to false positive and false negative rates. Depending on the availability, expertise and cost, a CT scan is more valuable. Other pituitary lesions are less common in reproductive medicine. A classic example, albeit rare nowadays, is pituitary apoplexy, or Sheehan's syndrome, following severe postpartum hemorrhage. Since thyrotropin-releasing hormone (TRH) and certain drugs can stimulate prolactin secretion, it is important to exclude primary hypothyroidism with a serum TSH measurement and a careful drug history prior to subjecting these patients to unnecessary investigations. Once hyperprolactinemia and any underlying organic causes have been excluded, ovulation is induced with pulsatile GnRH or gonadotropin therapy.

Elevated Serum FSH. Rarely, primary ovarian failure is a reason for amenorrhea in a young woman of reproductive age. These women may have symptoms of hot flashes and other manifestations of low endogenous estrogen as described earlier. Investigation includes serial serum FSH levels to ensure that the elevated postmenopausal levels are persistent. Karyotyping will be necessary to exclude Turner's syndrome (the mosaic form) in which menstrual function may be present in the early reproductive years and the florid features of classic Turner's syndrome are absent. Other investigations are directed at screening for an autoimmune cause. Ovarian failure following chemotherapy, radiotherapy, and surgery for systemic disease or malignancy will be obvious from the history. The impact of environmental toxicants, including toxic metabolites of cigarette smoke on ovarian failure, remains to be evaluated. With respect to infertility treatment, various regimens have been suggested but remain anecdotal. These include the use of gonadotropin stimulation (a) with or without prior suppression of gonadotropin levels with estrogen and progestogen replacement or GnRH agonists[13] and (b) with high-dose corticosteroid suppression of potential immunological factors contributing to ovarian failure.[1,4] A more realistic and successful method is the use of donor oocytes. This involves the synchronization of the patient's endometrium with ovarian steroids and the transfer of embryos derived from successful insemination of donor oocytes with sperm from the patient's partner. Potential limitations are the availability of donor oocytes, the cost and emotional stress involved, and the legal and ethical issues surrounding this approach.

Tubal/Pelvic Factors

Peritubal adhesions are commonly due to previous pelvic inflammatory disease (PID) or endometriosis. Tubal blockage is usually the sequelae of PID except for previous voluntary tubal sterilization. Another cause of tubal blockage is prior resection of part of the fallopian tube for a tubal pregnancy.

Previous PID

Classically, gonorrhea is the culprit for infertility due to tubal disease. It is now well recognized that PID is frequently polymicrobial. In addition, subclinical chlamydial infection may cause irreparable tubal damage. While mycoplasma has been implicated, it has not been proven to be a cause. Empirical treatment with doxycycline has been suggested if this organism is identified on a routine bacteriologic culture. PID can be silent or nonspecific even during the active phase, as in the case of chlamydial infection. Thus, while a prior history of documented PID is informative, infertile women frequently might not even know that they had the infection until during the infertility work-up. Investigation includes a HSG and a diagnostic laparoscopy. Depending on the site(s) and extent of the disease, surgical treatment or in vitro fertilization and embryo transfer (IVF-ET) will be the options. In addition, the type of adhesions or tubal blockage will dictate whether an operative laparoscopy or a conventional laparotomy is performed. With the recent availability of better-designed laparoscopic instruments and laser technology, adhesiolysis and salpingostomy can be successfully performed with laparoscopy to reduce the postoperative morbidity and hospital cost associated with conventional laparatomy. The prognosis for pregnancy is relatively good if pelvic adhesion alone is the major contributing factor. In this case, adhesiolysis (ovariolysis, salpingolysis) will be appropriate.

The location of tubal blockage is described as proximal, mid-segment, or distal with respect to the fallopian tube.[11] In general, the prognosis for pregnancy is best following microsurgical reversal of tubal sterilization, with overall live birth rates varying from 60–80%. The results, of course, are dependent on the type of sterilization procedure and the expertise of the surgeons. In the case of tubal re-anastomosis following a mid-segment resection for a tubal pregnancy, the prognosis for pregnancy will depend on factors that caused the initial ectopic pregnancy and the tubal and pelvic status subsequent to removal of the ectopic pregnancy. Distal disease varies from bilateral fimbrial agglutination to florid hydrosalpinges. Depending on the clinical picture, the surgical approach is fimbrioplasty and/or salpingostomy. Frequently, the pregnancy rate does not match the tubal patency rate, reflecting intrinsic mucosal and fimbrial tubal damage. Conventionally, proximal blockage is dealt with by microsurgical re-anastomosis of the intramural (interstitial) portion of the fallopian tube with the patent tubal section distally after excising the blocked segment. In selected cases, the transcervical approach to unblock the interstitial portion of the fallopian tube under a combination of hysteroscopic, radiographic, or ultrasound guidance may be successful. However, this should only be considered if underlying causes such as an intramural fibroid distorting the proximal tubal segment and concomitant mid-segment or distal disease have been excluded. Prior to tubal surgery, patients should be counseled with respect to the success rates, the alternatives, such as IVF-ET, and be warned of increased ectopic rates should pregnancy occur.

ENDOMETRIOSIS

While it is generally accepted that infertility can be attributed to endometriosis associated with anatomical distortion or damage of the fallopian tubes and ovaries and/or in the presence of adhesion formation, controversy exists concerning the relationship between minimal and mild endometriosis and infertility.[14] Definitive diagnosis can be made only by direct visualization at laparoscopy and, if necessary, combined with biopsies of suspicious, atypical areas. Depending on the age of the patient, symptoms (infertility versus pelvic pain), and the stage of the disease, treatment is initiated accordingly either by medical suppression (danazol, GnRH agonist, or progestogen), conservative surgery, or a combination of both. Pelvic adhesions and a large ovarian endometrioma do not respond to medical suppression. In addition, because of the side effects and contraceptive action of medical suppression, and the lack of definitive evidence that medical treatment of endometriosis improves fertility, conservative surgery (if possible, by operative laparoscopy) is usually more appropriate if infertility is the main concern. Whether to use cautery or laser to ablate foci of endometriosis depends more on the availability of equipment and expertise of the surgeons than on one having a distinct advantage over the other. In patients who fail conventional treatment for endometriosis, gamete intrafallopian transfer (GIFT) or IVF-ET is an alternative.

Uterine Factors

The diagnosis of uterine fibroids does not necessarily equate with infertility or recurrent abortion. In fact, the majority of women with uterine fibroids do not have any problem conceiving. In some instances, however, the size and location of the fibroid(s) may cause anatomical distortion of tubo-ovarian relationship or proximal tubal blockage. Rarely, a large submucous fibroid may occupy a substantial area of the intrauterine cavity, which may affect embryo implantation. It is important to exclude other factors that may contribute to infertility prior to considering surgery. The effect of Asherman's syndrome or uterine synechiae has been discussed earlier. Uterine anomalies of the septate or bicornuate type generally do not affect fertility but have been associated with recurrent abortion. Diagnosis of uterine factors is made by a HSG and hysteroscopy. Excision of a submucous fibroid or a septum can be performed at the time of hysteroscopy.

Cervical Factors

Cervical mucus containing antisperm antibodies or of poor quality and/or low quantity have been implicated to interfere with sperm-mucus interaction and, hence, fertility. The postcoital test is used to screen for these factors. While this test is very simple in theory, controversy surrounds the performance of the test with respect to coitus, the correlation of an abnormal test, the detection of antisperm antibodies, and subsequent pregnancy outcome.[9] If cervicitis is suspected to cause an abnormal postcoital test, empirical antibiotic treatment can be tried because a specific microbe is rarely incriminated. Previously, estrogen supplementation has been tried in an effort to increase cervical mucus. It is now more common to undergo intrauterine insemination to bypass the cervix.

Immunologic Factors and Unexplained Infertility

While immunologic factors may play a role in infertility, a sensitive and specific test that can predict infertility is lacking. In the absence of a specific therapy, treatment remains empirical, such as intrauterine insemination with washed sperm. Systemic illnesses that affect general health, menstrual function, and loss of libido are obvious contributing factors to infertility, and treatment is directed at the underlying problems. Similarly, sexual dysfunctions of psychogenic origin such as vaginismus or impotence require appropriate psychological counseling and treatment. There remain 10–15% of couples who have no factors that can be attributed to the infertility; these cases are labeled as unexplained. In such patients, 3–4 cycles of controlled ovarian hyperstimulation with gonadotropins combined with intrauterine insemination have been recommended prior to undergoing GIFT/IVF-ET.[6]

RECURRENT LOSS OF PREGNANCY

Acute management of a pregnancy loss involves an accurate diagnosis and, depending on gestational age, a curettage to remove the products of conception to arrest bleeding and alleviate discomfort. Patients with three consecutive first trimester spontaneous abortions or one midtrimester abortion require evaluation for an underlying cause. Major causes are chromosomal abnormalities, uterine defects, incompetent cervical os, and endocrine abnormalities, including inadequate luteal phase function. Other causes that have been proposed include infectious agents, autoimmune disease, parental immunologic compatibility, and environmental toxins.[2] Hence, investigation includes karyotyping of both partners to exclude a balanced chromosomal translocation and a HSG with or without hysteroscopy to exclude uterine anomalies. If an incompetent cervix is suspected, careful follow-up during pregnancy is recommended. If appropriate, a cervical cerclage is inserted to arrest further cervical dilatation in the absence of uterine contractions. A serum TSH level is used to screen for hypothyroidism. Luteal phase defect is evaluated by a well-timed midluteal phase serum progesterone level and a late luteal endometrial biopsy. A mycoplasma culture of the endometrium is also recommended. Autoimmune screening (circulating anticardiolipin antibodies and lupus anticoagulant) is undertaken to exclude lupus erythematosus. If lupus erythematosus is present, patients are treated with prednisone and low-dose aspirin throughout pregnancy. Parental sharing of histocompatibility antigens has been observed in some couples with recurrent abortion. This is detected by typing the human leukocyte antigens (HLA) of both partners. One immunologic treatment being evaluated is vaccination of the female with the partner's leukocytes. At this stage, this treatment modality should be considered experimental, and potential side effects remain unknown. Thus, HLA typing should not be routine. Despite these investigational recommendations, the yield of a positive test is, in general, low. Women should be advised to decrease cigarette smoking and alcohol use. Exposure to other toxicants and pregnancy loss remains to be critically assessed. It is also important to note that psychological support alone may lead to a marked improvement in pregnancy outcome (86%) if no abnormal findings are identified.[12]

ANTENATAL DIAGNOSIS

In couples at high risk of producing offspring with genetic disorders, preconception genetic counseling is important. However, detection of sporadic cases of birth defects in couples considered to be of low risk remains problematic. Morphologic abnormalities such as neural tube defects (NTD) can be detected by high-resolution ultrasound. Detection of genetic disorders and birth defects involves some of the following methods: ultrasonographic evaluation targeted at fetal morphologic abnormalities; amniocentesis or chorionic villus biopsy for detection of genetic disorders; amniocentesis for detection of markers of congenital defects in amniotic fluid such as α-fetoprotein for NTD; fetal echocardiography for fetal cardiac anomalies; fetoscopy for fetal blood sampling, direct fetal visualization and biopsy; and percutaneous umbilical blood sampling. The latter provides a means for karyotyping of fetal blood, detecting congenital infection with IgM titers, analyzing enzymes for specific deficiencies that are lethal, and providing ABO, Rh, and other antigen status. Details of these methods, including the risks and benefits of each, are available in most standard postgraduate textbooks of obstetrics. Recently, preimplantation genetic diagnosis has been attempted in which preembryo biopsy is performed in combination with IVF-ET and DNA technology. In the absence of the lethal genetic disease, the biopsied embryos are transferred as in routine IVF.[8] Important limitations are the potential ethical and legal consequences of this approach, the costs and emotional stress involved, and the suboptimal pregnancy success rate after embryo transfer during routine IVF. Preconception prevention of birth defects will be the ultimate goal. Prior to conceiving, women with a preexisting disease such as diabetes mellitus should consult their physicians to ensure that their condition is under optimal control. Physicians should review all medications used in terms of their potential teratogenic effects and switch to safer alternatives, if appropriate. Preconception modification of social behaviors such as heavy cigarette and alcohol consumption will minimize fetal exposure of these harmful substances and prevent low birthweight and prematurity associated with smoking and fetal alcohol syndrome. The use of vitamin supplements (folic acid) during the periconception period has been recommended to prevent NTD.[7]

REFERENCES

1. Blumenfeld Z, Halachmi S, Peretz BA, et al: Premature ovarian failure—the prognostic application of autoimmunity on conception after ovulation induction. Fertil Steril 59:750–755, 1993.
2. Carson SA (ed): Non-genetic causes of spontaneous abortions. Semin Reprod Endocrinol 7:103–197, 1989.
3. Cheung AP, Chang RJ: Polycystic ovary syndrome. Clin Obstet Gynecol 33:655–667, 1990.
4. Corenblum B, Rowe T, Taylor P: High-dose, short-term glucocorticoids for the treatment of infertility resulting from premature ovarian failure. Fertil Steril 59:988–991, 1993.
5. Cramer DW, Walker AM, Schiff I: Statistical methods in evaluating the outcome of infertility therapy. Fertil Steril 32:80–86, 1979.
6. Dodson WC, Whitesides DB, Hughes CL, et al: Superovulation with intrauterine insemination in the treatment of infertility: A possible alternative to gamete intrafallopian transfer and in vitro fertilization. Fertil Steril 48:441–445, 1987.
7. Folic acid and neural-tube defects—time for action? [editorial]. N Engl J Med 327:1875, 1992.
8. Hardy K, Martin KL, Leese HJ, et al: Human preimplantation development in vitro is not adversely affected by biopsy at the 8-cell stage. Hum Reprod 5:708–714, 1990.
9. Moghissi KS: Sperm-cervical mucus interaction. In Keel BA, Webster BW (eds): Handbook of Laboratory Diagnosis and Treatment of Infertility. Boca Raton, FL, CRC, 1990, pp 149–165.
10. New MI, Lorenzen F, Lerner AJ, et al: Genotyping steroid 21-hydroxylase deficiency: Hormonal reference data. J Clin Endocrinol Metab 57:320–326, 1983.
11. Sotrel G: Tubal Reconstructive Surgery. Philadelphia, Lea & Febiger, 1990.
12. Stray-Pedersen B, Stray-Pedersen S: Etiologic factors and subsequent reproductive performance in 195 couples with a prior history of habitual abortion. Am J Obstet Gynecol 148:140–146, 1984.
13. Surrey ES, Cedars MI: The effect of gonadotropin suppression on the induction of ovulation in premature ovarian failure patients. Fertil Steril 52:36–41, 1989.
14. Thomas EJ: Endometriosis and infertility: A continuing debate. In Shaw RW (ed): Advances in Reproductive Endocrinology—Endometriosis, Vol 1. Park Ridge, NJ, Parthenon, 1990, pp 107–117.

B. L. LASLEY, PhD
SUSAN E. SHIDELER, PhD

METHODS FOR EVALUATING REPRODUCTIVE HEALTH OF WOMEN

From the Division of
  Reproductive Biology
School of Medicine
  and Institute of Toxicology
  and Environmental Health
University of California
Davis, California

Reprint requests to:
B. L. Lasley, PhD
Division of Reproductive
  Biology
School of Medicine
  and Institute of Toxicology
  and Environmental Health
University of California
Davis, CA 95616

The previous chapter has described in detail the endpoints used for assessing the reproductive health of women. The approach taken there was from a clinical perspective, which may not be useful for most nonclinical settings. Many of the events of importance to female reproductive health occur without the awareness of women or their physicians; however, these events also cannot be evaluated through questionnaire or interview in the nonclinical or field setting. Ovulation, implantation, and luteal function can only be assessed through examination of tissue or hormone assays of blood or urine. Thus, some type of biological sampling is required to evaluate reproductive function accurately. Physical examinations, biopsies, and even the collection of opportunistic blood samples generally are not appropriate, practical, or ethical in most large field study designs. This kind of sampling is not possible outside a clinic and most likely not justifiable outside clinical fertility evaluations. Nonetheless, there is a growing need to develop ways to evaluate all aspects of women's reproductive health outside the clinic. This chapter will largely focus on the use of urine assays in the assessment of reproductive health.

More women of childbearing potential are entering the industrial and agricultural work force each year and are exposed to new chemical and physical agents that are being produced at a rate that outdistances our ability to screen them properly. The combination of these two elements leads to an increasing public concern that environmental factors could contribute to an apparently growing trend in infertility among young women.[17] It has been estimated that as much as 37% of the infertility in women younger than 24 has some link to reproductive toxic exposure.[17] Pregnancy failure is frequently examined for adverse reproductive health effects as a result of environmental exposures because early fetal development is considered most vulnerable to chemical insults. Early pregnancy loss has been correlated to chemical exposures.[20] Reduced fertility also may be a sensitive indicator of other health risks separate from failure of early pregnancy. For example, when fertility is impaired as a result of decreased ovarian function, it is likely that other aspects of women's health are also at risk as a consequence of decreased sex steroid production: Decreased bone deposition in the second and third decade of life[6] and increased risk of cardiovascular disease[15] are two examples of pathologies attributable to chronic decreased ovarian function.

Currently there is a need to identify and develop methods that permit the collection and assessment of both personal exposure information as well as biological samples from nonclinical populations. Clearly, the need for medical histories and screening interviews are critical to permit the selection of well-defined patients and the identification of reproductive abnormalities that would confound the interpretation of the results. The present approach to meeting these needs is to conduct entry interviews at the initiation of a study, to provide a streamlined log for daily exposure and menstrual information, and to have each patient collect her own urine samples daily.

Over the past 10 or 20 years, urine has become the biological sample of choice in nonclinical settings because urinary assays have become increasingly acceptable as methods for evaluating reproductive health.[12] Urine sampling has the advantage of being self-collectable and noninvasive, and samples are easily stored and transported. Assays for ovarian, pituitary, and trophoblastic hormone metabolites have been adapted to urine and formatted into economical assays that are ideal for epidemiologic studies.[16] The primary benefits of these urinary assays are that they permit daily samples to be collected for prolonged times with a high degree of compliance among nonclinical-based populations. In addition, most hormone metabolites in urine are found in relatively high concentrations. Hence, direct assay of the diluted urine is possible, thereby eliminating costly and time-consuming extraction procedures required for serum evaluations.

This is not to imply that urine samples can be used in place of blood samples or provide the same information at a reduction of time and money. Instead, urine samples provide a related but different kind of information, and specific limitations and concerns are associated with them. For example, it is necessary to recognize that variations in a patient's hydration level will be reflected in variations in urinary output throughout the day, and this can affect the concentrations of hormone metabolites measured in samples. As long as these limitations are understood and considered in each study design, the advantages of urinary monitoring far outweigh any disadvantages. Recently, large population-based studies have been conducted in which tens of thousands of urine samples were collected from hundreds of women.[7,22] While there is still need for improvement of some of the analytical methods, the overall results from these studies appear to be reliable and show that the approach holds promise for future applications.

The remainder of this chapter will focus on the use of urine samples in specific assay systems that are directed toward monitoring female reproductive health in population-based studies. The emphasis will be on recent developments in this area with an effort to discuss the strengths and weaknesses of each approach.

URINARY ASSAYS TO DETECT EARLY FETAL LOSS

Urinary assays have been employed since the early 1980s to detect early fetal loss (EFL) and, principally, the transient rise of immunoreactive human chorionic gonadotropin (hCG) in urine was used to recognize losses. The very wide range of results that have been published since the early 1980s reflects the variety of assay methods used, the demographics of the study populations, differences in the definition of early fetal loss, and differences in analytic methods.[12] While laboratory methods have improved markedly over the past 20 years, there has been much less progress in increasing our understanding of the expected frequency of EFLs in unexposed populations or in defining the characteristics that constitute either the events themselves or the physiologic mechanisms associated with them. It is remarkable that no standard definition for an "early fetal loss" exists, even today. Known pregnancies that are lost are generally considered to be clinical spontaneous abortions, but the very early loss of the products of conception not known to the woman is considered to be an "occult" or early loss. This kind of arbitrary definition makes review of the literature difficult and generalizations impossible regarding frequencies of "very early" or "occult" losses versus later clinical spontaneous abortions.

While many previous studies of early fetal loss suffered from limitations of assay sensitivity and specificity, technological improvements in these areas have not resolved all of the issues relating to these studies.[11] Under ideal conditions, and assuming normal fecundability, at least three or four ovulatory menstrual cycles with exposure to pregnancy must be studied in order to observe one conception. Hundreds or thousands of episodes of unprotected intercourse around the time of ovulation must be studied in order to calculate a population frequency of pregnancy loss with confidence. Some studies have limited the collection of urine to the time that the initiation of all pregnancies would be observed, but other studies have collected samples every day in order to completely characterize each menstrual cycle and accurately define each ovulatory cycle.[7,12,22] While the former approach has clear economic advantages, the data discussed below suggest that the latter approach is required despite its additional costs.

Most likely, the collection of daily urine samples for analysis with a highly specific and ultra-sensitive immunoradiometric assay, as performed by Wilcox et al.,[27] is the ideal strategy for assessing EFL. However, this approach is prohibitively expensive when the experimental design generates tens or hundreds of thousands of samples. Alternately, Taylor et al.[25] attempted to combine a highly sensitive, economical "screening" assay with a more specific "definitive" assay for hCG to solve this economic problem. Samples were screened initially with a highly sensitive, but less specific, enzyme immunometric assay that permitted as many as one third of the samples with no detectable hCG concentrations to be omitted from subsequent analysis. Samples determined to exhibit some hCG activity by the screening assay were then evaluated with the definitive radioimmunometric assay.

In contrast to the prevailing view of 10 years ago, the current understanding is that hCG is not a unique substance produced only by the trophoblast. Convincing data have demonstrated that hCG is secreted by the pituitary of normal nonpregnant women[19] and that secretion can be accelerated by gonadotropin-releasing hormone (GnRH).[18] It is not uncommon to observe elevations of immunoreactive hCG immediately following the midcycle gonadotropin surge in urine samples. Thus, the presence of elevated hCG alone can no longer be considered definitive evidence that a conceptus is present. Whether the earlier misconception that hCG was the definitive test contributed to some of the higher estimates of early loss rates is not yet known, but present knowledge negates the idea that pregnancies can be detected simply by the presence of detectable levels of hCG. Thus, the absolute sensitivity and specificity of assays for hCG alone may not be as important as once believed for detecting pregnancies.

Current approaches to detecting early pregnancies employ at least four additional criteria: threshold elevations of hCG above a detection limit, duration of the hCG elevation, timing, and association of the hCG elevations with ovulation. The setting of the threshold limit for hCG detection requires the establishment of a "basal" level of urinary hCG that is detected by the assay in women who are not exposed to pregnancy—often women with bilateral tubal ligations—but who are similar to the study population in most other aspects.[22,27] Their level of urinary hCG is used to establish the upper limit of pituitary hCG excretion and the threshold for hCG detection of a pregnancy. Since single-day spikes of pituitary hCG can be relatively high, a duration criteria is added in order to avoid false positives or having to set the threshold so high that a large number of rises of truly trophoblastic hCG are excluded. Concentrations of hCG are generally required to be above the threshold value for 2 of 3 or 3 of 4 consecutive days to eliminate single-day, pituitary-derived hCG spikes from creating false positives while preserving the utility of the highly sensitive assay.[11,22,27] Whether concentrations of hCG need to be indexed by creatinine (Cr) to adjust for difference in urine concentration has not been resolved. Since the rise of hCG is usually very rapid and the difference in urine concentration between days is usually small, it could be argued that the minor adjustment provided from creatinine would also be small and therefore unnecessary.

Since the elevation of pituitary-derived, urinary hCG following the midcycle gonadotropin surge can be elevated for several days and can fulfill the criteria of threshold and duration, the criteria of timing also is required in order to assure that the periovulatory interval is avoided. This, in turn, requires the identification of the periovulatory samples by additional hormone assays, assuming that samples were collected throughout most, if not all, of every menstrual cycle. Baird et al.[1] used the ratio of urinary estrogen and progesterone metabolites to identify the "transition days," and Clough et al.[4] proposed the use of an assay to detect the midcycle gonadotropin surge through the measurement of the intact LH and free alpha subunit of LH in daily urine samples. Both methods are highly reliable in detecting the periovulatory period in ovulatory cycles, and both permit the identification of the "window" of possible detection of hCG from an implanting embryo as distinct from pituitary-derived hCG spikes. Limiting the detection threshold rules to the appropriate window as described above eliminates concerns regarding the generation of false positives as a result of pituitary-derived hCG associated with the midcycle gonadotropin surge.

URINARY ASSAYS TO MONITOR OVARIAN FUNCTION

The use of urinary assays to measure ovarian steroids and assess ovarian function has lagged behind the use of urinary hCG for detecting early pregnancy.

Part of the reason for the slower acceptance of urinary assays for ovarian hormone evaluations has been the technical limitations, but the main reason is a lack of confidence that measurements of ovarian steroid metabolites in urine provide an accurate assessment of ovarian function.

Steroids are the principal ovarian hormones and are not aqueous-soluble. They are transported in the vascular bed, bound to large protein molecules such as sex-hormone binding protein and albumin. The primary ovarian steroids, estradiol and progesterone, are metabolized by the liver and then conjugated to either glucuronic acid or sulfate to form aqueous-soluble forms that are easily excreted by the kidney. A great deal of variation is found between species and even between individuals in the processes of conjugation and reabsorption of steroids by the gut. Large differences between individuals are found in the amount of steroid excreted in urine and passed through the gut, and urinary excretion varies greatly between individuals even when difference in urine volume or concentration are considered and compensated for by indexing with creatinine measurements. Even though mean or composite profiles illustrate the parallelism between blood and urine concentrations, it is difficult to establish absolute limits for normal and abnormal urinary steroid metabolite concentrations that can be applied to all individuals. This inability to use "fixed" concentration thresholds limits the interpretation of urinary steroid metabolite profiles at the present time to the major ovarian events that can be determined by relative changes in metabolite excretion rate.

Despite the fact that steroid conjugates are concentrated many-fold in urine, the fact that they have altered primary structures and are conjugated to glucuronic acid or sulfate makes them undetectable with conventional assays used to measure the circulating parent steroid. The advent of antibodies to the principal conjugates, i.e., estrone glucuronide and pregnanediol-3-glucuronide, opened the door to explore and take advantage of urinary monitoring of ovarian hormone production. Enzyme-based assays now exist for both estradiol and progesterone metabolites, and these assays have been applied to studies involving thousands of menstrual cycles.

A number of reports published over the past 8 years provide descriptions of reliable and economical assay methods and demonstrate that these methods can provide accurate assessments when applied properly.[1] In the near future, several additional studies will be published in which daily urine samples and paired blood samples have been analyzed. Furthermore, thousands of menstrual cycles have already been analyzed for ovarian steroid metabolites for large population-based studies, and the data from these analyses also will be published soon. These reports will provide the first comprehensive investigations in which ovarian function, determined by urinary hormone analyses, will have been compared within and between women and will undoubtedly usher in a new era in monitoring ovarian function and determining aberrations in such function in relation to occupational exposures. Taken together, these combined studies will demonstrate how broadly urinary data can be used and dispel lingering doubts regarding the utility of this approach.

A very strong dogma that menstrual calendars were accurate retrospective assessments of ovarian function existed for decades.[26] Regular, episodic vaginal bleeding was accepted as reasonable and sufficient proof that all components of ovarian function were therefore "normal." Over the past 20 years, however, our understanding of ovarian function has progressed to the point that we no longer make a direct or causative association between vaginal bleeding and specific aspects of ovarian function. We hesitate to define the "normal" menstrual cycle for lack of a "gold standard" for comparison. We now recognize that a great deal of variation in ovarian function can be associated with relatively regular menstrual calendars and that individual cycles should be evaluated by daily hormone measurements in order to understand the basis for observed variations in length of cycle.

Population-based studies are extremely difficult, if not impossible, to conduct when repetitive blood samples are required for any reason. The evaluation of serial or even periodic ovarian cycles would be impossible if self-collected urine samples were not the biological sample used to monitor daily hormone dynamics. The ability to have subjects collect and freeze their own daily urine samples for several consecutive menstrual cycles for laboratory analysis of ovarian steroids permits the study and characterization of normal and abnormal menstrual cycles with an emphasis on the temporal aspects of the environmental factors that contribute to each.

While daily samples may not be necessary to document the occurrence of major ovarian events, such as ovulation and luteal function, it is clear that the closer one approximates daily sampling, the more comprehensive and accurate the assessment of ovarian function becomes. While a single blood or urine sample in the last half of the intermenstrual interval can confirm that ovulation occurred, identification of the day of ovulation or determination of the length of the follicular and/or luteal phase to determine delay of ovulation or adequacy of the luteal phase requires daily, or near daily, sampling. Virtually all of the comprehensive descriptions of human menstrual cycles in standard texts depict daily concentrations of circulating hormones that required the collection of daily blood samples from individual women.[28] It is not surprising, therefore, that there are no detailed descriptions of consecutive menstrual cycles in the older literature since even the most highly motivated patient hesitates to continue a study requiring more than one month of daily venipunctures. Consequently, we know of no data sets with serum values documenting ovarian function in repetitive menstrual cycles and, yet, the evaluation of repetitive cycles is what is required to assess occupational and/or environmental effects on ovarian function.

Progesterone Metabolites

The primary urinary metabolite of progesterone is pregnanediol-3-glucuronide (PdG), and, in normal women, this metabolite exceeds 5 μmol per day during the luteal phase of the menstrual cycle when the daily production rate of progesterone is 10 μg or more. Thus, 15–30% of all progesterone is metabolized and excreted in the urine as PdG in concentrations that are easily measured during the luteal phase.[8] The daily profile of urinary PdG, particularly when individual samples are indexed by creatinine, when compared to analyses of paired serum samples, parallel serum progesterone profiles with a 1–3 day lag.[16] PdG rises relatively soon after ovulation and tends to lag behind the rise in serum progesterone by 1 or 2 days. The decline of PdG is generally much slower than that of serum progesterone and may still be returning to the basal levels 4 or 5 days after the onset of the menstrual period.

Based on analyses of paired urine and blood samples, when elevated PdG concentrations (more than 3 or 4 μg/mg Cr) immediately precede vaginal bleeding and decline during the menstrual period, one can almost always be assured that a luteal phase has been documented. The fact that no absolute upper or lower concentration of PdG has been established for detecting luteal function, however, should warn against overextending the interpretation of PdG measurements. While detecting the luteal phase by measuring daily PdG concentrations in urine has been reported many times,[3,14,21] and while this is not considered to be problematic, the use of PdG measurements for assessments beyond the documentation of a luteal phase should be done with caution and with consideration of the rather wide variation in excretion rates.

Despite the strong dogma suggesting that PdG excretion is a reliable indicator of progesterone production, recent data would suggest that more than the expected amount of variation in excretion exists between women. Most validation studies have focused on luteal phase levels of PdG and compared these measurements to measures of circulating levels of progesterone during this period. Since progesterone concentrations are 20–50 times higher in the luteal compared to the follicular phase,[28] and since concentrations are notoriously variable due to episodic pituitary luteinizing hormone pulses,[4] the mean elevation of urinary PdG during the composite luteal phase of several ovulatory menstrual cycles has been taken as a confirmation of the close association of serum progesterone and urinary PdG.[16] When follicular phase concentrations of urinary PdG were compared to the relatively constant circulating follicular phase concentrations, however, the results were not as comforting. It became clear that as much as a 10-fold difference exists between women with respect to progesterone metabolism and excretion when appraised by urinary PdG.[3] These data provide strong evidence that absolute PdG concentrations, regardless of whether they are indexed for urine volume or concentration differences, may not provide uniform information for different women and perhaps not even for different cycles within the same woman.

The fact that urinary PdG evaluations do not necessarily provide the same kind of information as serum measurements does not mean that urinary PdG measurements cannot or should not be used to monitor luteal function. For the most part, elevations of PdG above 3 or 4 μg/mg Cr for 3 or 4 days is indicative of a luteal phase, particularly when daily samples have been analyzed, peak concentrations of PdG precede the next menstrual period, and the decline of PdG concentrations coincide with the next menstrual period. Levels below these absolute levels in an ovulatory menstrual cycle, however, can lead to cycles being misidentified by the same criteria. In order to ensure against misclassification of ovulatory cycles of women with low PdG excretion patterns, increments of PdG excretion above the follicular phase baseline for that same cycle should be calculated and examined. Ovulation can be completely ruled out only when follicular phase baseline levels of PdG do not double for 3 or 4 days prior to the next episode of vaginal bleeding. When this approach is taken, it is possible to distinguish between ovulatory and anovulatory intermenstrual intervals consistently.[9]

Estrogen Metabolites

While several reports demonstrate the ability of urinary measurements of estrogen metabolites to accurately monitor ovulation and implantation, this technology has not been broadly applied. The reasons for this are fourfold: (1) the lack of consensus as to which estrogen metabolite best reflects serum estradiol, (2) the low signal-to-noise ratio of the estrogen profile throughout most of the menstrual cycle, (3) the limit of useful reagents with which to develop assays, and (4) the lack of convincing data that urinary estrogen profiles provide useful information beyond that provided by PdG and hCG for ovulation and EFL, respectively. As discussed below, these problems largely have been resolved, and it is likely that the measurement of urinary estrogen metabolites will become as common and as useful as PdG measurements in the future.

The overriding limitation of using urinary estrogen metabolites to monitor ovarian function in the past has been the combination of the low signal-to-noise ratio and/or the relatively narrow range of values observed through the normal menstrual cycle. HCG and PdG concentrations range 10-fold or more from nadir to peak in association with the physiologic events they reflect. In contrast, estrogen metabolites reveal only a threefold to fivefold increase above baseline during the normal menstrual cycle. This lower signal-to-noise ratio (or total range of concentrations) make indexing estrogen measurements to compensate for differences in urine volume or concentrations essential. If the full range of estrogen concentrations are fourfold from the early follicular phase to the preovulatory peak and if the urine concentrations can range twofold or more, it is easy to see that the physiologic profile could be obscured by unrecognized fluctuations in urine volume. Creatinine is a useful but imperfect compensator for urine concentration differences, and urine volume fluctuations remain a concern in tracking estrogen excretion in early morning urine samples.

The lack of consensus regarding which urinary metabolite of serum estradiol is most informative arises from a single report in which several estrogen metabolites were measured simultaneously.[10] In terms of the relation of each individual metabolite to the serum estradiol peak, estradiol glucuronide was the apparent best metabolite, with estrone glucuronide a close second. The concentration of estradiol glucuronide, however, was less than that of estrone glucuronide. The higher concentration of estrone glucuronide, as well as the availability of antibodies for this metabolite, made estrone glucuronide the practical choice in early studies.[11] Some workers selected antisera that cross-reacted to both estrone glucuronide and estrone sulfate because these conjugates exhibited parallel profiles and their combined measure increased the signal to noise ratio.[23] For practical reasons, the measurement of estrone glucuronide, or the combined measure of both estrone conjugates, will be the prevailing choice, at least for the immediate future.

Beyond these technical issues, the important questions remaining are: What unique physiologic information is provided by urinary estrogen metabolites that is not provided by other biomarkers, and does the information justify the effort? At least four kinds of information appear to be provided by the measurement of urinary estrogens: (1) follicular dynamics, (2) prediction of ovulation, (3) day of ovulation, and (4) confirmation of implantation. Since the day of ovulation is addressed below in the context of the midcycle gonadotropin surge and since implantation is traditionally detected with hCG, the focus here will be on detecting follicular dynamics and predicting ovulation.

A few reports have been published that compared paired serum estradiol and urinary estrone conjugate measurements and demonstrated parallelism between the mean profiles of the two measures.[16] The urinary profile lags behind the serum estradiol by slightly less than one day, and urinary dynamics are dampened by about 20% compared to serum dynamics. The concentration of serum estradiol, however, is often near the limit of detection in normal women and often below the limit of detection in amenorrheic or oligomenorrheic women. Thus, much of follicular dynamics are not reliably detected by serum estradiol prior to the development of the dominant follicle in the mid- to late follicular phase of the ovulatory menstrual cycle. In contrast to serum, the concentrating effect of the kidney on steroid metabolites makes the detection of low-level estrogen dynamics easier in urine. This difference, together with the need to collect serial blood samples to follow follicular dynamics, makes monitoring of ovarian follicles by urine superior to serum techniques when longitudinal measurements are necessary. Studies of perimenarchial girls and perimenopausal women demonstrate this point.[5,14]

Despite the lag time and attenuation of the urinary measures of estrogen metabolites compared to serum estradiol, the two measures were found to be comparable in predicting ovulation in a study evaluating a limited number of normal menstrual cycles.[24] This single study suggests that daily early morning urine samples can be used to measure the initiation of the preovulatory estrogen rise and to predict the ovulatory event by 3–5 cycle days. Potential false positives due to developing follicles regressing rather than ovulating were avoided by selecting women with normal length, ovulatory menstrual cycles.[13] Nonetheless, this study showed that it is possible to detect follicular events and anticipate ovulation with only early morning urine samples. The reliability of urinary estrone conjugates to predict ovulation accurately also has been demonstrated in monkeys by the increased conception rate of rhesus monkeys that were bred according to the preovulatory urinary estrogen conjugate rise.[2]

URINARY ASSAYS TO MONITOR PITUITARY FUNCTION

The measurement of intact LH and FSH in urine is still acceptable even though there are legitimate concerns regarding the dissociation of the subunits in frozen-thawed urine samples.[1] Theoretically, the integrated measure of urinary LH would be superior to that of serum LH because the effects of pulsatility , or missing the LH surge by evaluating a single serum sample, would be absent in the urinary measure. This superiority has not been realized due to the high degree of metabolism of the intact dimer prior to excretion in urine. Use of FSH measures have been hampered by the lack of a direct assay for urinary FSH, which would end the need for acetone precipitation and eliminate some errors resulting from differential recovery.

A novel strategy for measuring the intact LH as well as the free alpha subunit has been developed to remove concerns regarding dissociation due to freeze-thaw and to amplify the midcycle gonadotropin surge has been developed.[4] This strategy consists of a simple enzyme assay that has been shown to be more than 95% effective in detecting the midcycle gonadotropin surge and in identifying the day of ovulation using only first morning urine samples. No parallel strategy for FSH has yet been reported.

SUMMARY

The use of urine as a practical sample for evaluating the reproductive health of women in population-based studies is still being developed and applied. The adaptation of enzyme-based assays for the assessment of ovarian steroids as well as simple computer algorithms for interpreting the data both simplify and increase the efficiency of modern reproductive epidemiologic studies. New statistical approaches and new assays have extended physiologic monitoring to include early pregnancy, luteal phase function, and ovulation. While urine is superior to blood sampling, it is important to remember, however, the limitations of urinary hormone measurements when applying them alone to identify specific types of reproductive failure because variations in metabolism and excretion rate still contribute some uncontrollable variation. The rate of progress in developing and refining these methods over the past 5 years indicates that urinary methods of reproductive monitoring will continue to dominate this field and eventually be used in the clinic as well.

REFERENCES

1. Baird DD, Weinberg CR, Wilcox AJ, et al: Using the ratio of urinary oestrogen and progesterone metabolites to estimate day of ovulation. Stat Med 10:255–266, 1991.
2. Behboodi E, Katz DF, Overstreet JW, et al: The use of urinary estrone conjugate assay for detection of optimal mating time in the cynomolgus macaque. J Med Primatol 20:229–234, 1991.
3. Branch CM, Collins PO, Kilpatrick MJ, et al: The effect of conception on the concentration of urinary oestrone-3-glucuronide, LH/hCG and pregnanediol-3-glucuronide. Acta Endocrinol (Copenh) 93:228–233, 1980.
4. Clough KM, Cole FX, Seaver SS, et al: Enzyme immunoassay method for total alpha gonadotropin in human urine samples. Fertil Steril 57:1241–1246, 1992.
5. DeVane GW, Soto D, Lasley BL: Daily urinary estrogen and progesterone metabolites at the time of menarche [abstract]. Society for Gynecologic Investigation, Phoenix, March 1985.
6. Fabbri G, Petraglia F, Segre A, et al: Reduced spinal bone density in young women with amenorrhoea. Eur J Obstet Gynecol Reprod Biol 41:117–122, 1991.
7. Gray RH, Corn M, Cohen R, et al: Final report. The Johns Hopkins University retrospective and prospective studies of reproductive health among IBM employees in semiconductor manufacturing. Baltimore, Johns Hopkins, May 1993.
8. Harkness RA, Davidson DW, Strong JA: The metabolism of small and large amounts of progesterone in man. Acta Endocrinol (Copenh) 60:221–236, 1969.
9. Kassam A, Overstreet JW, Gold EB, Lasley BL: A simple algorithm using daily urinary pregnanediol-3-glucuronide to evaluate luteal phase progesterone production [abstract]. Society for the Study of Gynecological Investigation, Chicago, March 22–25, 1994.
10. Knobil E: The neuroendocrine control of the menstrual cycle. Recent Prog Horm Res 36:53–79, 1980.
11. Lasley BL, Gold EB, Nakajima ST, et al: Misclassification of adverse reproductive effects can be minimized by measurements of multiple biomarkers for ovarian toxicity and early fetal loss. In Proceedings of Hanford Symposium on Health and the Environment. J Toxicol Environ Health 40:423–433, 1993.
12. Lasley BL, Mobed K, Gold EB: The use of urinary hormonal assessments in human studies. Ann N Y Acad Sci 709:299–311, 1994.
13. Lasley BL, Shideler SE, Munro CJ: A prototype for ovulation detection: Pros and cons. Am J Obstet Gynecol 165:2003–2007, 1991.
14. Lasley BL, Stabenfeldt GH, Overstreet JW, et al: Urinary hormone levels at the time of ovulation and implantation. Fertil Steril 43:861–867, 1985.
15. Matthews KA, Bromberger J, Egeland G: Behavioral antecedents and consequences of the menopause. In Korenman SG (ed): The Menopause. Norwell, MA, Serono Symposia, USA, 1990, pp 1–10.
16. Munro CJ, Stabenfeldt GH, Overstreet JW, et al: Serum and urinary ovarian steroids assessed by RIA and EIA. Clin Chem 37:838–844, 1991.
17. National Research Council: Biomarkers in Reproductive Toxicology. Washington, DC, National Academy Press, 1989.
18. O'Dell WD, Griffin J: Pulsatile secretion of chorionic gonadotropin during the normal menstrual cycle. J Clin Endocrinol Metab 69:528–532, 1989.
19. O'Dell WD, Griffin J: Pulsatile secretion of human chorionic gonadotropin in normal adults. N Engl J Med 317:1688–1691, 1987.
20. Pastides H, Calabrese EJ, Hosmer DW Jr, et al: Spontaneous abortion and general illness symptoms among semiconductor manufacturers. J Occup Med 30:543–551, 1988.
21. Prior JC, Vigna YM, Schechter MT, et al: Spinal bone loss and ovulatory disturbances. N Engl J Med 323:1221–1227, 1990.
22. Schenker MB, Beaumont J, Eskenazi B, et al: Final report to the Semiconductor Industry Association: Epidemiologic study of reproductive and other health effects among workers employed in the manufacture of semiconductors. Final Report, Davis, CA, University of California Davis, December 1992.

23. Shideler SE, Czekala NM, Kasman LH, et al: Monitoring ovulation and implantation in the lion-tailed macaque (Macaca silenus) through urinary estrone conjugate evaluations. Biol Reprod 29:905–911, 1983.
24. Shideler SE, DeVane GW, Kalra PS, et al: Ovarian-pituitary interactions during the perimenopause. Maturitas 11:331–339, 1989.
25. Taylor CA, Overstreet JW, Samuels SJ, et al: Prospective assessment of early fetal loss using an immunoenzymometric screening assay for detection of urinary human chorionic gonadotropin. Fertil Steril 57:1220–1224, 1992.
26. Treloar AE, Boynton RE, Behn BG, et al: Variation of the human menstrual cycle through reproductive life. Int J Fertil 12:77–126, 1967.
27. Wilcox AJ, Weinberg CR, O'Connor JF, et al: Incidence of early loss of pregnancy. N Engl J Med 319:189–194, 1988.
28. Yen SSC, Jaffe RB: Reproductive Endocrinology. 3rd ed. Philadelphia, WB Saunders, 1991.

ELLEN B. GOLD, PhD
ELIZABETH TOMICH, BS

OCCUPATIONAL HAZARDS TO FERTILITY AND PREGNANCY OUTCOME

From the Division of Occupational/
Environmental Medicine and
Epidemiology
School of Medicine
and Institute of Toxicology
and Environmental Health
University of California
Davis, California

Reprint requests to:
Ellen B. Gold, PhD
Associate Professor
Division of Occupational/
Environmental Medicine and
Epidemiology
Institute of Toxicology
and Environmental Health
University of California
Davis, CA 95616

Supported by a Research Career
Development Award from the Na-
tional Institute of Environmental
Health Sciences, 5 K04 ES00202-4
(EBG).

Fertility can be measured by a number of indices. These include menstrual function (regularity of cycles, cycle length, characteristics of bleeding), ovarian function (magnitude and timing of secretion of ovarian steroids and pituitary gonadotropins), fecundability ratios (to express probability of conception as ratios of observed to expected conceptions, accounting for the number of menstrual cycles followed and, often, contraception and frequency of intercourse) and time to conception (as measures of subfertility). Progress of pregnancy and pregnancy outcome can be assessed by hypertension, threatened abortion, preeclampsia (as measures of pregnancy complications), preterm labor, prematurity, low birthweight, small size for gestational age, spontaneous abortion, and still-birth. However, for few of these indicators are records routinely collected and available, and virtually for none of these indicators are such records obtained in the occupational setting. In addition, some of the indicators do not require medical attention, which means that many affected women do not seek care and that use of medical records to determine the frequency of these outcomes will result in underestimation. Further, many of these outcome indicators are not readily accessible to investigators to measure or monitor in occupational epidemiologic studies of reproductive hazards in the workplace, thus making such studies logistically difficult and expensive. Thus, it is perhaps not completely surprising that relatively little research has been conducted for many of these outcomes and that most of the research that has been conducted has focused on the more readily observed or assessed outcomes, such as pregnancy loss and birthweight.

Fertility, gestation, and pregnancy outcome are in turn dependent on a number of biologic processes, including semen function and quality, function of the hypothalamic-pituitary-ovarian axis, and normal cell division and differentiation in the developing fetus. Disruption of any of the many biologic processes or the organs responsible for them by occupational exposures will increase the risk of subfertility or infertility, adverse pregnancy progress and outcome,[4] and congenital malformations or childhood cancer. Many of these biologic processes, as well as effects of occupational exposures on risk of congenital malformations and childhood cancer, are discussed elsewhere in this volume and will not be discussed here.

FERTILITY

Methodologic Issues in Studying Subfertility or Infertility

A number of indicators of fertility can be monitored or measured in epidemiologic studies of putative occupational reproductive hazards. These most often include indicators of the fertility of the couple, such as the clinical definition of one year of unprotected intercourse without clinical evidence of pregnancy,[6,71] the ratio of observed to expected births (standardized fertility ratio),[45,97] and time (usually months or menstrual cycles) to pregnancy.[3] All of these focus on the fertility of the couple rather than on the biologic processes contributing to fertility.[6] The clinical definition provides a dichotomous outcome, which has desirable properties for analysis (although generally requiring a larger sample size) but loses information about the continuous nature of the probability of conception.[4] The standardized fertility ratio provides a readily interpretable number to assess risk, but it is relatively insensitive,[6] depends on knowledge about the expected number of births based on a population that is comparable in age and parity to the one being observed, requires information on the use of contraception,[6] and requires relatively large populations to detect moderately reduced fertility.[25] Time to conception provides a more sensitive measure of the nature of fertility[6] and, while permitting control of confounding variables, also reflects the fact that interference with any of the many biologic processes required for conception will increase the time to achieve pregnancy, particularly for low-dose exposures, without necessarily resulting in frank infertility. However, this indicator only examines pregnancies and how long it takes to achieve them and does not include women who never become pregnant. This indicator is also more difficult to measure, because it requires collection of accurate data on the number of menstrual cycles until pregnancy occurs and on confounding variables that might affect fertility, such as frequency of intercourse, use of contraceptives, and other exposures to reproductive toxicants or risk factors for infertility.

Some studies have focused on the effect of occupational exposures on male biologic processes that may contribute to infertility, and these are discussed in chapter 5. A few, particularly recent, studies have focused on indicators of adverse effects of occupational exposure on female biologic processes that may affect fertility, such as menstrual cycle length and variability,[20] which are indirect measures of ovulatory function,[28] or directly measured ovarian function.[24] The methodologic issues that arise in these types of studies have been reviewed previously[9,39,85] and include using as the unit of observation the woman or the menstrual cycle, the number of cycles contributed in a fixed time being inversely related to a woman's cycle length and variability, the need for inclusion of a large number of cycles, the dependence of variations in observations of cycle length on the nature of the population studied, and the insensitivity of menstrual cycle length and variability to disturbances in ovarian function.

In addition, when considering an exposure of interest, one must also consider the study design and how it might influence the findings. For example, cross-sectional studies that examine history of infertility or subfertility or menstrual disorders consider only workers who are currently working in the exposed and comparison occupations with respect to such reproductive history, but they do not consider women who may have left such occupations either because of the effects on their reproductive health or for other reasons. Thus, historical cohort studies are better designed to minimize such concerns, but many involve recall of long-past menstrual cycles, contraception, and patterns of intercourse. Case-control studies also generally involve recall of past (potentially long ago) events but often have the advantage of observing more cases than historical or prospective cohort studies. However, by design, case-control studies compare multiple possible occupations and exposures, which makes validation of exposures difficult (if not impossible) and raises the distinct possibility that some risk estimates will be statistically significant by chance alone due to the large number of occupations or exposures that are being compared. Further, case definitions and selection of comparison groups must be carefully considered so as to minimize potential biases.[44] In addition, cohort or case-control studies must pay careful attention to potential confounding factors such as age, educational level, smoking, and consumption of alcohol and caffeine.[3,35,37,64,93] Failure to examine and control for the effects of confounding factors can produce biased results and inconsistencies between studies that have seemingly investigated very similar exposures and outcomes. In the reviews of each of the studies presented in this chapter, potential confounders that were considered by the authors—even if they were found not to affect the results, as well as ones that did—will be presented. Such design issues must be carefully considered when reviewing the results of studies, particularly when they seem inconsistent.

Occupational exposures associated with risks of compromising the three measures of a couple's fertility discussed above were reviewed in *Occupational Medicine: State of the Art Reviews* in 1986 by Baird and Wilcox.[4] In this chapter, only an update of the literature since 1986 for these outcomes will be provided, as well as a review of studies that examined the effect of occupational exposures on menstrual cycle function.

Occupational Exposures and Risk of Altered Menstrual Cycle Function

Several occupational exposures associated with menstrual disorders have recently been catalogued.[6] Some of the earliest studies of adverse effects of occupational exposures on menstrual cycle function were conducted by investigators in the former Soviet Union.[42] They compared 302 women ages 20–40 who worked in a superphosphate manufacturing plant where they were exposed to dust containing **fluoride** to 309 office workers and housewives. The exposed women were five to six times more likely to have irregular menstruation, with the risk increasing with dust exposure, and four times as likely as controls to have inflammation of the uterus, cervix, and vagina.

Women with high exposure to **toluene** have been reported recently to have increased *and* decreased frequency and severity of dysmenorrhea compared to community controls, but no differences have been observed for workers with low exposure, or in frequency of irregular cycles, long cycles, or increased duration or amount of menstrual bleeding.[59] In the Netherlands, significantly higher frequencies of dry cleaning workers exposed to **perchloroethylene** reported unusual cycle lengths (fewer than 26 or more than 30 days), menorrhagia, dysmenorrhea, and premenstrual syndrome compared to laundry workers.[101] In addition, a recent report indicates that hairdressers, who are exposed to a number of chemical agents that may affect the hypothalamic-pituitary-ovarian axis as well as physical stressors, had significantly higher frequencies of irregular cycles, unusual cycle lengths, oligomenorrhea, long menstrual bleeding, and more severe and longer lasting menstrual pain than a comparison group of shop assistants. The statistically significant risk estimates ranged from 2.4 to 9.4.[8] Amenorrhea was also increased in hairdressers, with a risk estimate of 6.5 (95% CI = 0.9–47.6).

Ovarian dysfunction in women occupationally exposed to **mercury** has also been reported from the former Soviet Union.[67] A recently completed study of women working in the manufacture of silicon wafers compared to women working in nonfabrication areas in the semiconductor industry in the United States also has revealed significantly increased menstrual cycle length and variability (as measured by the standard deviation in cycle length) in women who work in thin film/ion implant activities,[21] which may involve exposure to **metal** dopants such as arsenic, which are used to alter the conductive properties of the wafers. In addition, significantly increased menstrual cycle variability was observed in women working in photolithography, which involves potential exposure to **organic solvents** such as xylene, n-butyl acetate, and glycol ethers.

In Italy, women in a lamp factory who were exposed both to **mercury** and to the stress of **noise** and **shift work** have been reported to have a higher incidence and prevalence of oligomenorrhea (cycles longer than 31 days) and changes in their menstrual cycles than workers in a comparison lamp factory who had stress factors but no exposure to mercury.[11] Risk of irregular cycles and amenorrhea recently have been observed to be significantly increased in women who work in slaughterhouses compared to those who work in canneries, the former having much greater likelihood to be working under the stress of **cold temperatures** and **irregular work schedules**.[57] Irregular schedules were also associated with an increased risk of having menstrual cycles longer than 32 days, but standing, assembly line work, handling weights regularly, and overall job satisfaction were not associated with irregular or long cycles or amenorrhea.[57]

The **stress** of being a new student, which could be considered to be an occupational exposure, has been reported to be associated both with shortened (fewer than 25 days[51]) and lengthened (longer than 43 days[26]) menstrual cycles. In the former study, the shortened cycle lengths were related to anovulatory cycles; longer cycles were associated with delayed ovulation.[51]

Occupational Exposures Associated with Reduced Fertility

Inability to conceive or to conceive within 1 year at some time during a couple's reproductive history has been estimated to occur in the population at a rate of 10–35%[66,71] and has been shown to be inversely associated with age and educational level. A number of the occupational exposures that have been associated with infertility or hormonal imbalance have recently been catalogued.[6]

One of the earliest occupational case-control epidemiologic studies of infertility examined several exposures in cases who were hospitalized (an unusual circumstance) for infertility of at least one year's duration. **Textile dye, lubricating oils, dry cleaning chemicals, metals** (such as those for welding, lead, cadmium, mercury) and **noise** were significantly associated with infertility and/or delayed conception[71] (Table 1). More recently, delay to conception (or reduced fecundability ratio) has been significantly associated with exposure to **antibiotics** in pharmacy assistants[80] and to **nitrous oxide** in dental assistants.[75] In addition, a study of female workers involved in the manufacture of silicon wafers in the semiconductor industry has shown a nonsignificant reduction in fecundability ratios among women working in areas of fabrication rooms that have exposure to **metal** dopants that are used to alter the conductive properties of the wafers.[16]

SPONTANEOUS ABORTIONS

Methodologic Issues

Perhaps because of its emotional impact, one of the largest areas of interest in research on occupational reproductive hazards has been the risk of spontaneous abortions (SAB). The large number of published reports in recent years are summarized in Table 2. A number of methodologic difficulties, however, arise in obtaining accurate measurement of the effect of occupational exposures on this reproductive outcome. First, cross-sectional, case-control, and historical cohort studies have the potential for recall bias, namely the potential for women with spontaneous abortions (in case-control and cross-sectional studies) to recall prior exposures better than women with normal pregnancy outcomes or for women with occupational exposures believed to be hazardous to recall pregnancy losses better than nonexposed women (in historical cohort studies). There is, however, some evidence[7] that this problem may not be a large one, particularly in historical cohort studies, since women do tend to recall SAB fairly accurately. Prospective cohort studies may overcome some of these limitations and are a feasible way to study SAB, which is not a rare occurrence in pregnancy. However, the prospective cohort design requires careful screening of large numbers of women (to identify women with opportunity for conception) since most women do not become pregnant in a given period of time and therefore may require lengthly follow-up, making this design very resource intensive.

A second methodologic concern is that pregnancies that are lost even before being recognized by the woman or her clinician will be missed. While this is certainly true in cross-sectional, case-control, and historical cohort studies, it is not clear if these losses would necessarily be more related to occupational exposures (and thus occur differentially in exposed and nonexposed groups) than recognized losses. Further, recent technological advances have made it possible to detect such losses in prospective cohort studies,[93] but such measurement increases costs of the study significantly. Two prospective studies of several hundred women with opportunity for pregnancy who were employed in the manufacture of silicon wafers in the semiconductor industry[15,24] have employed these new techniques, with estimated costs for each study in the millions of dollars.

Potential selection bias is another methodologic difficulty of a number of the studies reviewed below, which look at the relation of occupational exposures to risk of SAB. Many of the studies only include current workers in an industry and examine the relation of past exposures to past pregnancy outcomes. Thus, in a

TABLE 1. Occupational Exposures and Risk of Subfertility or Infertility: Review of Studies

Reference	Design	Number of Cases; Age Range	Type of Cases/Outcome	Comparison Group	Source of Exposure Information	Findings (95% Confidence Interval)	Potential Confounders Considered
Rachootin and Olsen[71]	Case-control	1,069; 21–46	Hospitalized for infertility of at least one year's duration	Parents of a healthy child conceived within one year	Job title, type of company, duties and exposures of couple from woman's questionnaire	OR = 5.2 (2.3, 11.5) for IFI and textile dye exp.; OR = 3.4 (1.2, 10.1) for IFI and exp. to cutting, lubricating oils; OR = 2.7 (1.0, 7.1) for IFI and DC and female exp. to dry cleaning chemicals or metal welding; OR = 2.6 (1.1, 5.9) for IFI and exp. to lead, cadmium, mercury; OR = 2.5 (1.1, 5.7) for DC and female exp. to antirust agents; OR = 2.4 (1.2, 4.9) for DC and male textile dye exp.; for consistency; OR = 2.2 (1.3, 3.9) for IFI and noise; OR = 2.1 (1.4, 3.2) for female hormone disturbance and exp. to noise; OR = 1.9 (1.5, 2.6) for DC and male heat or to female exp. to noise or plastic manufacturing; OR = 1.7 (1.0, 2.8) for DC and female exp. to lead, mercury, cadmium; OR = 1.3 (1.0, 1.7) for DC and male metal welding or noise	Woman's age, education, residence, parity, smoking, drinking, past use of oral contraceptives

Study	Design	Population	Outcome	Comparison group	Exposure measurement	Results	Confounders
de Rosis et al.[11]	Cross-sectional	26; all ages	One year of unprotected intercourse without conception	Lamp factory workers with no mercury exposure but some stress factors	Measurement of mercury exposure and questionnaire	OR = 1.21 for primary subfecundity in mercury lamp factory workers	None
Schaumburg and Olsen[80]	Historical cohort	2,557 pregnancies; all ages	Time to pregnancy in union of pharmacy assistants	Pharmacy assistants with administrative and counter jobs	Questionnaire	No significant association with specific pharmacy assistant jobs; OR = 1.34 (1.0–1.8) for exp. to antibiotics and > 12 month wait to pregnancy	Age, parity, smoking, alcohol consumption
Rowland et al.[75]	Cross-sectional with retrospective information on pregnancies	418 women with pregnancies; 18–39	Time to pregnancy in dental assistants	Dental assistants unexposed to nitrous oxide	Occupational exp. asked on phone interviews	FR = 0.94 (0.90–0.98) for each hour of exp. to unscavenged nitrous oxide per week; FR = 0.41 (0.23–0.74) for ≥ 5 hours/week of exp. to unscavenged nitrous oxide; Longer mean time to conception for high unscavenged exp. to nitrous oxide	Age, race, smoking, history of pelvic inflammatory disease, frequency of intercourse, number of sexual partners, recent use of oral contraceptives

DC = delayed conception; FR = fecundability ratio; IFI = infertility; OR = odds ratio

TABLE 2. Studies of Occupational Exposures and Risk of Spontaneous Abortions

Reference	Age Range	Study Design	Study Subjects — Cases/Exposed Group	Study Subjects — Comparison Group	Source of Exposure Information	Findings (95% Confidence Interval Unless Otherwise Noted)	Potential Confounders Considered
Electromagnetic Fields/Microwaves/VDTs							
Juutilainen, Matilainen, Saarikoski, et al.[38]	All ages	Case-control	Early pregnancy loss determined by serum human chorionic gonadotrophin	Women with normal pregnancies (n = 102)	Measurements of extra low frequency radiation magnetic fields in homes and workplace, job classification from questionnaire about occupation.	OR = 1.15 (0.3, 4.7) for early pregnancy loss and occupational magnetic field exp.; OR = 5.09 (1.0–26) for early pregnancy loss and magnetic field ≥ 0.63 μT at front door of residence; OR = 4.65 (0.9–25) for early pregnancy loss and mean magnetic field of residence ≥ 0.25 μT	Maternal age, residence, maternal smoking, type of dwelling, SES, occupation
Ouellet-Hellstrom, Stewart[65]	All ages	Nested case-control	All recognized miscarriages in female members of American Physical Therapy Association with known gestational age	All pregnancies except ectopic, matched on maternal age at conception and time from conception to questionnaire completion	Self-administered questionnaire	OR = 1.28 (1.02–1.59) for SAB and using microwave diathermy during pregnancy; OR = 1.50 (1.04–2.17) for SAB and using microwave diathermy 5–20 times/month; OR = 1.59 (0.99–2.55) for SAB and using microwave diathermy > 20 times/month; OR = 1.07 (0.91–1.24) for SAB and using microwave diathermy; OR = 1.10 (0.88–1.38) for SAB and using shortwave diathermy 5–20 times/month; OR = 0.87 (0.63–1.20) for SAB and using shortwave diathermy > 20 times/month	Maternal age, gravidity, time since last use of oral contraceptives, prior fetal losses, time from conception to interview, genitourinary conditions, smoking, use of electric blankets, water beds, heated mattress pads, and other treatment modalities

Reference	Age	Study design	Cases	Controls/Cohort	Method	Results	Confounders
Lindbohm, Hietanen, Kyyronen, et al.[47]	20–35	Case-control	Women employed as bank clerks and clerical workers who had a SAB	Women employed as bank clerks and clerical workers who gave birth and did not have a SAB or malformed infant during 1975–1985 (n = 394)	Mailed questionnaire on work history and use of VDTs in first trimester, company records on models of VDTs used, measurement of magnetic fields of VDTs	OR = 1.1 (0.7, 1.6) for SAB and use of VDT in first trimester; OR = 1.7 (0.9, 3.4) for SAB and 11–20 hrs/week VDT use; OR = 2.0 (0.8, 3.7) for SAB and > 20 hrs/week VDT use; OR = 3.4 (1.4, 8.6) for VDTs with magnetic field levels > 0.9 μT; Increasing risk with increasing hours × magnetic flux	Year of pregnancy, maternal age at conception, previous births, previous SAB, use of IUD, quantity of work, exp. to solvents, frequency of technical breakdowns, hrs. of use per week, mental workload, smoking, alcohol use, previous diseases
Roman, Beral, Pelerin, Hermon[74]	All ages	Case-control	Nulliparous working women with a clinically diagnosed SAB	Nulliparous working women attending antenatal care (n = 297)	Interview	Women working with VDUs are not at increased risk of SAB. Adjusted OR = 0.9 (0.6, 1.4) No trends in numbers of hours spent weekly on the VDU, tasks for which VDU used, or with passive VDU exposure	Age, previous SAB, type of employment, marital status, housing tenure, education, smoking, alcohol use, partner's occupation
Schnorr, Grajewski, Hornung, et al.[81]	18–33	Historical cohort	Married, full-time telephone operators who used VDTs at work (n = 323)	Married, full-time telephone operators who did not use VDTs at work (n = 407)	Company records, telephone interview, measurement of VDT EMF	OR = 0.93 (0.63, 1.38) for SAB and VDT use in first trimester; OR = 1.04 (0.61, 1.79) for SAB and weekly VDT use = 1–25 hrs; OR = 1.00 (0.61, 1.64) for SAB and weekly VDT use > 25 hrs; OR = 0.99 (0.68, 1.44) for all fetal loss and VDT use	Age, gravidity, race, education, current employment, years employed at company, previous SAB, smoking, thyroid disorder, alcohol consumption, physical stress, psychological stress

(Continued on next page)

TABLE 2. Studies of Occupational Exposures and Risk of Spontaneous Abortions (*Continued*)

Reference	Age Range	Study Design	Study Subjects		Source of Exposure Information	Findings (95% Confidence Interval Unless Otherwise Noted)	Potential Confounders Considered
			Cases/Exposed Group	Comparison Group			
Daniell, Vaughan, Millies[10]	All ages	Historical cohort	Flight attendants (n = 514)	1. Mothers employed outside the home (n = 264) 2. Other mothers, regardless of employment (n = 475)	Maternal usual occupation on birth certificate	RR = 1.9 (1.3, 2.7) for fetal loss in flight attendants compared to all controls; RR = 1.3 (0.9, 1.9) for fetal loss in flight attendants compared to employed controls	Paternal occupation, income, maternal employment, race, maternal chronic illness, maternal and paternal age, gravidity, parity, months since last pregnancy, prenatal care, marital status
Windham, Fenster, Swan, Neutra[95]	≥ 18	Case-control	Working residents of Santa Clara County, Calif. who had a SAB by 20 weeks gestation, last menstrual period in 1986	Working county residents who had a live birth	Telephone interview	OR = 1.2 (0.89, 1.7) for SAB and < 20 hrs. VDT use/week; OR = 1.2 (0.88, 1.6) for SAB and ≥ 20 hrs VDT use/week; OR = 1.4 (1.0, 2.0) for SAB and ≤ 12 weeks gestation and < 20 hrs. VDT use/week; OR = 1.3 (0.9, 1.8) for SAB and ≤ 12 weeks gestation and ≥ 20 hrs. VDT use/week; OR = 0.7 (0.4, 1.1) for SAB and > 12 weeks gestation and < 20 hrs. VDT use/week; OR = 0.9 (0.6, 1.4) for SAB and > 12 weeks and ≥ 20 hrs. VDT use/week	Employment status, maternal age, race, education, marital status, prior fetal loss, insurance for prenatal care, alcohol use, smoking, hospital, last menstrual period, number of hours worked, shift worked, time from last menstrual period to interview, quality of interview response, gestational age at SAB

Study	Age	Design	Cases	Comparison group	Method	Results	Adjustments
Goldhaber, Rolen, Hiatt[22]	> 17	Nested case-control	SAB in working women	Working women with live births	Phone interviews or mail questionnaires	Adj. OR = 1.8 (1.2–2.8) for VDT use > 20 hrs/wk. in first trimester	Age, previous SAB, race, education, smoking, alcohol, occupation gestational age at pregnancy diagnosis, hospital of delivery
McDonald, McDonald, Armstrong, et al.[53]	All ages	Cohort	Women employed for 30+ hrs./week at start of pregnancy and using VDU at work	1. All working women 2. All working women not using VDU	Nurse or telephone interview	*Relative to all working women* RR = 1.19 (90% CI 1.09, 1.30) for SAB and VDU use for current pregnancies, with dose-response for hours of use; RR = 0.97 (90% CI 0.89, 1.05) for SAB and VDU use for previous pregnancies *Relative to working women not using VDUs* RR = 1.06 (90% CI 0.8, 1.4) for SAB and VDU use for current pregnancies; RR = 1.01 (90% CI 0.7, 1.3) for SAB and VDU use for previous pregnacies	Age, gravidity, previous SAB, ethnicity, education, smoking, alcohol, year of conception
Nurminen, Kurppa[62]	All ages	Cohort	Women with symptoms of threatened abortion (bleeding) that were employed in office work	Women giving birth that were employed in non-office work	Interview, using job titles	No increased risk of threatened abortion for office workers Adj. RR = 0.8 (0.5–1.4)	Previous pregnancy, diseases, drugs, alcohol, smoking, working conditions, non-occupational exposure, frequency of VDT exposure, history of menstrual irregularity

(Continued on next page)

TABLE 2. Studies of Occupational Exposures and Risk of Spontaneous Abortions *(Continued)*

Reference	Age Range	Study Design	Study Subjects — Cases/Exposed Group	Study Subjects — Comparison Group	Source of Exposure Information	Findings (95% Confidence Interval Unless Otherwise Noted)	Potential Confounders Considered
Ericson, Kallen[13]	All ages	Cohort	Women hospitalized for SAB who worked in occupations with potential VDT exposure	National population of women giving birth	Occupation code from census information	O/E = 1.1 (90% CI 0.9, 1.2) for SAB and high VDT work; O/E = 1.0 (90% CI 0.8, 1.3) for SAB and medium VDT work; O/E = 0.9 (0.8, 1.1) for SAB and low VDT work	SES, maternal age, parity, delivery unit, county of residence
Wertheimer, Leeper[91]	All ages	Cross-sectional	Pregnant women using electric blankets or water beds	Pregnant women not using electric blankets on water beds	Phone interviews	Fetal loss rate = 6.8% in users of electric blankets or water beds, 4.2% in non-users, $p < 0.05$	None
Solvents							
Gray, Corn, Cohen, et al.[24]	20–44	Historical cohort	Pregnant clean room workers	Pregnant non-clean room workers in semiconductor industry	Interview and hygiene assessment	Adj. RR = 2.8 (1.4–5.6) for women working in previous group with ethylene glycol ethers	Age, year
Swan, Beaumont, Hammond, et al.[88]	18–44	Historical cohort	Pregnant women working in fabrication of silicon wafers	Pregnant women working in nonfabrication areas in semiconductor industry	Telephone interviews and industrial hygiene assessments	Adj. RR = 2.40 (1.24–4.11) for medium and high exposure scores for ethylene-based glycol ethers, with dose-response observed	Age, smoking, education, income, ethnicity, pregnancy history, year, stress

Study	Age	Design	Exposed group	Comparison group	Method	Results	Confounders
Ng, Foo, Yoong[59]	All ages	Cross-sectional	Women specifically exposed to high concentration of toluene (50–150 ppm) working in an audio speaker factory who were married and had a pregnancy (n = 55)	1. Similar women working in the same factory but low exp. to toluene (0–25 ppm) (n = 31) 2. Women in the general community undergoing routine care at public maternity clinics (n = 190), 15% currently and 35% previously employed in factories	Personal interviews on occupational exps.	OR = 4.20 (1.01, 22.86) for SAB and high toluene exp. vs low exp.; OR = 2.79 (1.32, 5.88) for SAB and high toluene exp. vs clinic women; OR = 5.72 (1.14, 28.75) for SAB after employment vs pre-employment at factory with toluene exp.	Maternal age, gravidity, SES, health care, level of physical work, shift work, smoking, alcohol use, previous SAB, race, years in plant
Lipscomb, Fenster, Wrensch, et al.[48]	15–49	Cross-sectional and retrospective	Women pregnant who had occupational solvent exp. (n = 52)	Other pregnant women without solvent exp. (n = 986)	Job title, exposures, industry, work activity and months employed from interviews	OR = 3.34 (1.42, 7.81) for SAB and occupational solvent exp.; OR = 1.10 (0.33, 3.73) women in electronics work	IUD use, maternal age, prior SAB, ethnicity, smoking, alcohol consumption, geographic residence, employment during pregnancy, non-occupational solvent exp.

(Continued on next page)

TABLE 2. Studies of Occupational Exposures and Risk of Spontaneous Abortions *(Continued)*

Reference	Age Range	Study Design	Study Subjects — Cases/Exposed Group	Study Subjects — Comparison Group	Source of Exposure Information	Findings (95% Confidence Interval Unless Otherwise Noted)	Potential Confounders Considered
Pinney, Lemasters[69]	All ages	Cross-sectional and retrospective	Female employees of the semiconductor industry working in fabrication (n = 189) or nonfabrication who were chemically exposed (NFC) (n = 74)	Women working in nonfabrication who were not chemically exposed (NFNC) (n = 191)	Questionnaires for job title and job duty, categorized by industrial hygienists	OR = 1.62 (0.77, 3.39) for SAB in fabrication vs NFNC; OR = 2.00 (0.85, 4.71) for SAB in NFC vs NFNC; OR = 2.49 (1.10, 5.63) for SAB in salaried vs hourly workers; OR = 1.35 (0.31, 5.94) for stillbirth in fabrication vs NFNC; OR = 1.72 (0.29, 10.09) for stillbirth in NFC vs NFNC	Maternal age, education, work in salaried position for fabrication exp., race, alcohol consumption, smoking, diabetes, fever or vomiting during pregnancy, paternal chemical exp., gravidity, prior SAB, prior fetal loss, prior induced abortion, recall interval
Windham, Shusterman, Swan, et al.[94]	≥ 18	Case-control	Women with pathology-proven SAB by 20 weeks gestation (n = 626)	Women having live births living in the same county and matched on last menstrual period and hospital (n = 1300)	Interview for occupation, industry and occupational and non-occupational exposures	OR = 1.1 (0.77, 1.5) for SAB and use of any solvent; *Crude* OR = 4.7 (1.1, 21.1) for SAB and perchlorethylene; *Crude* OR = 3.1 (0.9, 10.4) for SAB and trichloroethylene; *Crude* OR = 2.3 (1.0, 5.1) for SAB and paint thinners; OR = 1.8 (1.1, 3.0) for SAB and aliphatic solvents; OR = 2.1 (0.64, 6.9) for SAB and paint strippers; No dose-response found for total hours exposed	Non-occupational solvent use, gravidity, maternal age, race, education, prior fetal loss, smoking, hours worked, alcohol and caffeine consumption, insurance, interview data quality, hospital, last menstrual period, marital status, prenatal care, separate solvent classes

Study	Age	Design	Population	Method	Results	Confounders
Lindbohm, Taskinen, Sallmen, Hemminki[46]	All ages	Nested case-control	Pregnant women biologically monitored for solvent exp. who had a SAB / Pregnant women biologically monitored for solvent exp. who did not have a SAB or malformed child (n = 167)	Questionnaires (job title and activities, solvents used), biological (urinary) exp. measurements, and industrial hygiene measurements	OR = 2.2 (1.2, 4.1) for SAB and occupational solvent exp.; OR = 2.1 (0.9, 5.1) for SAB and exp. to aliphatic hydrocarbons; OR = 3.9 (1.1, 14.2) for SAB and high exp. to aliphatic hydrocarbons; OR = 5.2 (1.3, 20.8) for SAB and graphic workers exp. to aliphatic hydrocarbons; OR = 9.3 (1.0, 84.7) for SAB and shoe workers exp. to toluene; OR = 3.4 (0.7, 16.9) for SAB and 1,1,1 trichloromethane exp.; OR = 2.7 (0.7, 11.2) for SAB and dry cleaning workers exposed to tetrachloroethylene; NSA for styrene, xylene and aromatic hydrocarbons in general and trichloroethylene	Maternal age, previous SAB, parity, smoking, alcohol use, fever diseases, lifting, exp. to other solvents
Ahlborg, Hogstedt, Bodin, Barany[1]	All ages	Prospective cohort	Women enrolling for prenatal care who were exposed during pregnancy to occupational stresses (chemical or physical) who worked as school teachers, social workers, nurses, lab workers, sales & service, hospitality, industrial workers, agric. workers / Office workers (no occupational exp. to chemical/physical stress)	Self-administered questionnaire	NSA of SAB risk with occupational solvent exp.	Maternal age, parity, sex of infant, previous SAB, education, passive & active smoking, alcohol use, coffee consumption

(Continued on next page)

TABLE 2. Studies of Occupational Exposures and Risk of Spontaneous Abortions *(Continued)*

Reference	Age Range	Study Design	Study Subjects — Cases/Exposed Group	Study Subjects — Comparison Group	Source of Exposure Information	Findings (95% Confidence Interval Unless Otherwise Noted)	Potential Confounders Considered
Taskinen, Anttila, Lindbohm, et al.[89]	18–40 (wives)	Case-control	Wives of workers monitored for organic solvent exp. who had a SAB (n = 120)	Wives of workers monitored for organic solvent exp. who had not had a SAB or a malformed child (n = 251)	Questionnaires to both spouses on occupation, work tasks and specific solvent exp. and biological monitoring of men (blood and urine) for specific solvents	OR = 2.3 (1.1, 5.0) for SAB and paternal exp. to organic solvents; OR = 2.6 (1.2, 5.9) for SAB and high/frequent exp. to organic solvents; OR = 2.3 (1.1, 4.7) for SAB and high/freq exp. to toluene; OR = 2.1 (1.1, 3.9) for SAB and high/frequent exp. to misc. organic solvents; OR = 3.3 (1.6, 6.8) for SAB in painters; OR = 3.8 (1.2, 11.9) for SAB in woodworkers	Maternal heavy lifting, history of previous SAB, maternal exp. to organic solvents, maternal smoking and alcohol consumption, paternal exp. to dusts, maternal age
Axelsson, Lutz, Rylander[2]	<44	Historical cohort	SAB verified in medical records for women working in a lab during their first trimester	Women not engaged in lab work during the first trimester of pregnancy	Questionnaire on jobs and solvent exposure; and job title from payroll records	Overall SAB Rate = 9.9% for lab workers *vs* 11.5% for non-lab workers; RR = 1.31 (0.89, 1.91) for lab workers exposed to organic solvents. (No dose-response relationship); RR = 3.2 (1.36, 7.47) for SAB with shiftwork during pregnancy. Highest SAB rate for self-reported exposure to formaldehyde (30%) and petroleum ether (28.6%) *p* = 0.02)	Maternal age, smoking, medication, infectious diseases during pregnancy, work with x-ray and radioactive isotopes, pregnancy number, year of pregnancy, previous SAB, shift work, work conditions, heavy lifting, stress

	Age	Design	Population	Exposure assessment	Results	Adjustments
Heidam[29]	18–40	Historical cohort	Women having SAB who were employed, including dental assistants, factory workers, gardening workers or painters	Postal questionnaire (self-reported)	Adj. OR = 1.7 (1.0, 2.9) for SAB in factory workers; Adj. OR = 2.9 (1.0, 8.8) for SAB in painters; NSA with organic solvents	Gravidity, pregnancy order, and maternal age
Heidam[30]	18–40	Historical cohort	Female lab workers exposed to chemicals in hospital labs and industrial labs (including university)	Self-reported occupational title and chemical exposure on postal questionnaire	NSA found for SAB in individual lab occupations; NSA found for SAB in lab workers exposed to specific chemicals	SES, gravidity, pregnancy order, maternal age
			Female workers *not* occupationally exposed to chemicals, including physiotherapists, occupational therapists, office workers, technical assistants and designers (n = 1431)			
Hydrocarbons McDonald, McDonald, Armstrong, et al.[52]	All ages	Historical cohort	Partners of women employed 30+ hrs./week at time of conception who had potentially harmful occupations	Father's job and industry from maternal questionnaire	O/E = 1.10 (90% CI 1.02, 1.20) for SAB and paternal mechanics, repairers, fabricators, and assemblers; O/E = 0.87 (90% CI 0.56, 1.29) for SAB and paternal occupations w/probable exp. to ionizing radiation; O/E = 1.21 (0.96, 1.49) for SAB and paternal physical scientists	Maternal age, gravidity, previous miscarriage, ethnic group, education, smoking and alcohol consumption, maternal occupation, previous pregnancies when not employed 30+ hrs./week
			Women employed 30+ hrs./week at time of conception and giving birth successfully			

(Continued on next page)

TABLE 2. Studies of Occupational Exposures and Risk of Spontaneous Abortions *(Continued)*

Reference	Age Range	Study Design	Study Subjects Cases/Exposed Group	Study Subjects Comparison Group	Source of Exposure Information	Findings (95% Confidence Interval Unless Otherwise Noted)	Potential Confounders Considered
Pesticides							
Restrepo, Munoz, Day, et al.[73]	All ages	Cross-sectional and retrospective	Women (n = 3490) or partners of men (n = 1594) working in the floriculture industry who had been pregnant	Pregnancies of the same workers prior to exp. to pesticides in floriculture	Interview on job category, pilot study to assess exp. to Captan (a fungicide), survey of companies for pesticide use patterns	OR = 2.20 (1.82–2.66) for SAB in female workers; OR = 1.79 (1.16–2.77) for SAB in wives of male workers; No trend in risk with size of company, amount of pesticides, or duration of work for SAB after exp.	Age at interview, age at pregnancy, pregnancy order, year pregnancy occurred, education, marital status
Heidam[29]	18–40	Historical cohort	Women having SAB who were employed, including dental assistants, factory workers, gardening workers or painters	Women giving birth who were employed in a less chemically exposed occupation during pregnancy	Postal questionnaire (self-reported)	Adj. OR = 1.3 (0.2, 7.1) for SAB in outdoor gardening workers; NSA for pesticides	Gravidity, pregnancy order, and maternal age
Electronics							
Beaumont, Swan, Hammond, et al.[7]	18–44	Historical cohort	Pregnant women working in fabrication of silicon wafers	Pregnant women working in nonfabrication areas in semiconductor industry	Telephone interviews and industrial hygiene assessments	Adj RR = 1.43 (0.95, 2.09) for SAB and fabrication; Adj. RR = 1.67 (1.04, 2.55) for SAB and photolithography; Adj RR = 2.08 (1.27, 3.19) for SAB and etching	Age, smoking, education, income, ethnicity, pregnancy history, year, stress

Reference	Age	Study design	Cases	Controls	Method	Results	Confounders
Shusterman, Windham, Fenster[86]	≥ 18	Case-control	Women having a pathology-proven SAB by 20 weeks gestation (n = 303)	Women who had live births, matched for hospital and last menstrual period (n = 655)	Questionnaire including exposure review by industrial hygienists and occupational physician	OR = 0.94 (0.58, 1.5) for SAB and any electronics production work; OR = 0.87 (0.45, 1.6) for SAB and semiconductor fabrication; OR = 1.1 (0.57, 2.2) for SAB and assembly work; OR = 0.96 (0.60, 1.5) for SAB and *all* electronics production; OR = 1.5 (0.62, 3.4) for SAB when performing > 2 steps in assembly; OR = 1.7 (0.38, 7.3) for SAB & diffusion step (within semiconductor fabrication); OR = 1.6 (0.29, 7.7) for SAB & encapsulation (assembly) OR = 1.4 (0.58, 3.4) for SAB & flux removal (assembly); OR = 1.3 (0.62, 2.7) for SAB & soldering (assembly) OR = 3.2 (0.47, 26.8) for SAB & exp. to potting compound (epoxy resin used in assembly)	Maternal age, ethnicity, education, smoking, alcohol consumption, previous SAB, hospital, last menstrual period, previous pregnancy history, physical stress (hours worked/week & hours stood/day), multiple exposure
Huel, Mergler, Bowler[36]	All ages	Cross-sectional and retrospective	Former micro-electronic assembly workers (n = 90)	Friends and relatives of workers not employed in micro-electronics industry (n = 90)	Self-administered questionnaire, company records	OR = 5.6 ($p < 0.01$) for SAB at start of employment; OR = 4.0 ($p < 0.05$) for SAB during employment	Ethnicity, maternal age, number of pregnancies before employment, education

(Continued on next page)

TABLE 2. Studies of Occupational Exposures and Risk of Spontaneous Abortions (*Continued*)

Reference	Age Range	Study Design	Study Subjects Cases/Exposed Group	Study Subjects Comparison Group	Source of Exposure Information	Findings (95% Confidence Interval Unless Otherwise Noted)	Potential Confounders Considered
Metals							
Ericson, Kallen[12]	All ages	Historical cohort	Dentists, dental assistants, and dental technicians (n = 1264)	Women with gainful occupations other than the dental field	Maternal occupation in census and birth registry	Dentists O/E = 1.10 for SAB Assistants O/E = 0.97 for SAB Technicians O/E = 1.36 for SAB	Maternal age, parity, year of birth, infant sex
McMichael, Vimpani, Robertson, et al.[56]	All ages	Prospective cohort	Pregnant women from Port Pirie (a lead smelting community) (n = 774)	Non-residents of Port Pirie	Questionnaire interview for occupation. Blood lead samples collected upon entering study (14–20 weeks), 32 weeks, at delivery and from umbilical cord	Mean blood lead = 11.3 ± 0.81 µg/dL in SAB, 10.8 ± 0.15 µg/dL in other pregnancies, NSA; Late fetal deaths = 17.5/1000 live births in Port Pirie vs 5.8/1000 in neighboring areas and 8.0/1000 in South Australia; NSA with mean blood lead in mid-pregnancy	Maternal age, years lived in Port Pirie, marital status, country of birth, race, blood pressure
de Rosis, Anastasio, Selvaggi, et al.[11]	All ages	Cross-sectional and retrospective	Women working in lamp factory and exposed to mercury (n = 153)	Lamp factory workers with no mercury exp. but some stress factors (n = 293)	Measurement of mercury exp. and questionnaire on history of exp.	OR = 0.72 for SAB in mercury lamp factory workers	Maternal age, employment duration, previous pregnancies, smoking, alcohol consumption

Hemminki, Niemi, Koskinen, Väinio[31]	15–39	Cohort	Members of Finnish metal workers' union having SAB	All Finnish women	Union registry and Industrial Health Staff	SAB rate union workers = 7.82/100 pregnancies vs 7.34/100 pregnancies in general population; SAB ratio union = 13.79/100 births vs 10.34/100 births in general population ($p < 0.001$); SAB rate for radio/TV manuf. (union) = 12.44 ($p < .01$); SAB ratio for radio/TV manuf. (union) = 20.87 ($p < .01$); SAB rate after joining union = 3.37 vs 5.71 before joining ($p < .001$); SAB ratio after joining union = 12.69 vs 10.16/100 births before joining ($p < .01$); SAB exp. to soldering in radio/TV manuf. = 41% vs 10% in general population	Age, reproductive history, occupation
Heidam[29]	18–40	Historical cohort	Women having SAB who were employed, including dental assistants, factory workers, gardening workers or painters	Women giving birth who were employed in a less chemically exposed occupation during pregnancy	Postal questionnaire (self-reported)	Adj. OR = 1.0 (0.6–1.6) for SAB among dental assistants; Significant association with nitrous oxide or inorganic mercury	Gravidity, pregnancy order, and maternal age

(Continued on next page)

TABLE 2. Studies of Occupational Exposures and Risk of Spontaneous Abortions *(Continued)*

Reference	Age Range	Study Design	Study Subjects Cases/Exposed Group	Study Subjects Comparison Group	Source of Exposure Information	Findings (95% Confidence Interval Unless Otherwise Noted)	Potential Confounders Considered
Medical Exposures							
Klebanoff, Shiono, Rhoads[40]	All ages	Historical cohort	Female medical residents who became pregnant (n = 1284)	Male physicians' non-physician spouses or mates who became pregnant (n = 1481)	Questionnaire	Hazard ratio = 1.13 (0.92, 1.40) for SAB in female residents vs spouses; Hazard ratio = 2.20 (1.21, 3.98) for SAB in anesthesiologists; Hazard ratio = 1.38 (0.92, 2.08) for surgeons, obstetricians, gynecologists vs. nonanesthetic-exposed specialties	Number of prior pregnancies, age, marital status, spouse in the medical field, medical specialization, smoking, race-ethnicity
McDonald, McDonald, Armstrong, et al.[54]	All ages	Cohort	Women working ≥ 30 hours at beginning of their pregnancy and hospitalized for SAB by < 28 weeks gestation	General population	Interviews by nurse, medical records	Nursing aides: O/E = 1.33 $p < .01$; Sales/services: O/E = 1.22 $p < .05$; Food/beverage service: O/E = 1.22 $p < .01$	Threatened abortion, age, gravidity, education, smoking, alcohol, ethnicity, weight, previous SAB
McDonald, Armstrong, Cherry, et al.[55]	All ages	Cohort	Women having SAB by < 28 weeks gestation	Women having term delivery	Hospital interviews/ phone interviews	Specific findings by nursing assistants for current pregnancy: O/E = 1.24, $p < .05$; for previous pregnancy: O/E = 1.13, $p < .05$ Specific findings by lab technicians for current pregnancy: O/E = 1.17 (90% CI = 0.8–1.6); for previous pregnancy: O/E = 0.94 (90% CI = 0.8–1.2)	Maternal age, parity, history of previous SAB, smoking, education

Reference	Age	Study design	Cases	Controls	Method	Results	Covariates
Selevan, Lindbohm, et al.[84]	≤ 40	Case-control	Female nurses working in areas of hospitals with high annual usage of antineoplastic drugs who had fetal loss (n = 124)	Female nurses without a recorded fetal loss working in hospitals using high amounts of antineoplastic drugs (n = 321)	Self-administered questionnaires on work history and occupational exp.	OR = 2.30 (1.20, 4.39) for SAB and exp. to antineoplastic drugs in first trimester; OR = 0.96 (0.36, 2.59) for SAB and exp. to anesthetic gases in first trimester; OR = 2.27 (0.94, 5.47) for SAB and exp. to x-rays in first trimester	Maternal age, smoking, alcohol use, health condition, medications used in first trimester, gravidity, prior fetal loss or induced abortion, contraceptive use, multi-drug exp. and year of pregnancy

Physical exertion

Reference	Age	Study design	Cases	Controls	Method	Results	Covariates
Florack, Zielhuis, Pellegrino, Rolland[19]	18–39	Cohort	Current hospital cleaners and kitchen staff who became pregnant	Current hospital clerical workers (n = 110) who became pregnant	Personal interview	Adj. OR = 1.07 (0.34–3.35) for SAB and at least one hour/day of lifting; Adj. OR = 3.19 (1.27–9.78) for SAB and at least one hour/day of bending; Adj. OR = 3.06 (1.06–8.85) for SAB and high peak abdominal pressure score; Adj. OR = 1.34 (0.44–4.01) for SAB and very high chronic abdominal pressure score	Age, gravidity, previous SAB, SAB in participants' mother, fertility treatments, medical drug use, current chronic disease, smoking, caffeine and alcohol consumption, education, occupational exposure
Nurminen[60]	All ages	Case-control	Women not giving birth to a child with malformations that had experienced a threatened abortion or pregnancy-induced hypertension and who worked ≥ 1 week the first trimester of their pregnancy	Mothers with normal pregnancies	Interviews 2–4 months after delivery	RR = 1.6 (1.0, 2.5) for threatened abortion and standing work compared to sedentary work; RR = 1.4 (0.8, 2.3) for threatened abortion and high short-term physical load; RR = 1.6 (1.0, 2.7) for hypertension and high short-term physical load in third trimester	Hospital region, maternal age, parity, outcome of previous pregnancies, smoking, alcohol use, drugs

(Continued on next page)

TABLE 2. Studies of Occupational Exposures and Risk of Spontaneous Abortions *(Continued)*

Reference	Age Range	Study Design	Study Subjects		Source of Exposure Information	Findings (95% Confidence Interval Unless Otherwise Noted)	Potential Confounders Considered
			Cases/Exposed Group	Comparison Group			
McDonald, Armstrong, Cherry, et al.[55]	All ages	Cohort	Women having SAB at <28 weeks gestation	Women having term delivery	Hospital interviews/ phone interviews	Specific findings for jobs with physical effort in service sector for current pregnancy: O/E = 1.58, p < 0.01; for previous pregnancy: O/E = 1.41, p < 0.01; Specific findings for jobs with physical effort in office sector for current pregnancy: O/E = 1.34, p < 0.05; for previous pregnancy: O/E = 1.44, p < 0.01; Specific findings for jobs with standing ≥ 6 hrs./day or 40 hrs./week working in manuf. for current pregnancy: O/E = 1.54–1.57, p < 0.01; for previous pregnancy: O/E = 1.03–1.06; Specific findings for jobs with heavy lifting in manuf. for current pregnancy: O/E = 1.43, p < 0.05; for previous pregnancy: O/E = 1.41, p < 0.01	Maternal age, parity, history of previous SAB, smoking, education

Adj. = adjusted; EMF = electromagnetic fields; IUD = intrauterine device; NFC = non-fabrication, chemically exposed; NFNC = non-fabrication, not chemically exposed; NSA = no significant association; O/E = observed/expected; OR = odds ratio; RR = relative risk; SAB = spontaneous abortion; SES = socioeconomic status; VDT = video display terminal; VDU = video display unit.

sense, only "survivors," or women who stayed in the industry, are being studied. The problem this potentially creates is that women who have had SAB may be more likely to continue employment while those who have given birth may be more likely to not return to work or may lose their jobs if parental leave is not provided. In some studies, this potential for bias is sometimes further accentuated by examination of current exposures among current workers in relation to past reproductive outcomes. This design not only raises the possibility of misclassification of exposure by assuming that current exposures accurately reflect those of the past, it also does not truly meet one of the criteria for deriving a causal inference: temporal sequence.[32] This relates to an additional exposure issue in such studies, namely that timing of exposure during gestation is critical to evaluating the relationship to relevant outcomes so that the typical dose-response criterion for deriving causal inferences also must take timing of exposure into consideration.[83]

Occupational Exposures Associated with Spontaneous Abortion

Studies of occupational hazards associated with risk of SAB have focused not only on chemical exposures but also on a number of physical exposures and psychological and physical stressors (*see* Table 2). Regarding **physical exposures**, several studies in the last decade have examined risks associated with occupational use of **video display terminals**; (VDTs) and electromagnetic field (EMF) and microwave exposure. Interest in risk of SAB associated with use of VDTs heightened with the publication of a paper by Goldhaber and colleagues in 1988[22] that showed an increased relative risk, particularly in women interviewed by telephone versus those who completed a mailed questionnaire. Most recent North American studies since then have reported no significant increase in risk of SAB associated with use of VDTs,[53,81,95] and some European studies also have shown no effect,[13,62,74] but others have shown a modest increased risk that is most notable when measurements of magnetic fields have been made.[47]

Interest in reproductive hazards associated with EMF exposure was aroused by Wertheimer's and Leeper's 1986 report that an increased risk of SAB was associated with use of electric blankets or water beds during the cold months[91] and a subsequent study by the same authors showing a different seasonal distribution of SAB but no difference in SAB rates in users and nonusers of ceiling cable electric heat.[91] A Scandinavian study found a significantly increased risk of early pregnancy loss associated with **residential magnetic field exposure** but not with maternal occupational magnetic field exposure.[38] An additional American study showed a modest but statistically significantly increased SAB risk associated with **microwave diathermy** use by physical therapists but no increased risk associated with shortwave diathermy.[65] In addition, a historical cohort study showed an increased risk of fetal loss among flight attendants,[10] which could be attributed to ozone exposure but also to other physical exposures such as radiation or physical stressors, including changes in time zones, disturbance in circadian rhythms and sleep patterns, or long hours standing and lifting. These factors are currently under study by the Industrywide Studies Branch of the National Institute for Occupational Safety and Health.

Many studies with cross-sectional, case-control, and historical cohort designs have found significantly increased risks of SAB in different occupational settings with maternal exposure to **organic solvents** in general,[89] but also for specific exposures ranging from **toluene**,[46,59,94] **perchlorethylene**,[94] **trichloroethylene**,[94] and glycol ethers[24,88] to **aliphatic hydrocarbons** in general.[46] The associations for glycol ethers have been observed most consistently.

A few studies also have reported a significantly increased risk of SAB in women working in **agricultural** settings[73] but have not been able to link the excess risk specifically to pesticides or other specific exposures. Goulet and Theriault[23] have reported a significantly increased risk of **stillbirth** in women with low level occupational exposure to **pesticides** or **germicides**, and McDonald and colleagues[54] also reported an elevation in risk of stillbirth for women working in agriculture and horticulture.

Several studies have examined the risk of SAB in **electronics** or **semiconductor** workers who are commonly exposed to low levels of organic solvents, and most have found an increased risk,[7,36] although not always statistically significant.[86] While some studies have observed no increased risks with exposure to organic solvents,[1] the findings of an association are largely consistent in studies of different designs, in different populations, and in different locations, and many have showed strong associations with large increases in risk. Of studies that have observed an overall increased risk of SAB with such exposures, a number have found no evidence of dose-response relationships,[94] but some have.[2,46,88] Thus, although the evidence may not be considered totally consistent and incontrovertible, it is strongly suggestive of a causal association for many of the organic solvents.

A few recent studies have focused on the relationship of various occupational **metal** exposures to risk of SAB. Largely no relationship has been found in recent studies with occupations that are likely to have exposure to **mercury** (dentists and dental assistants and technicians or lamp factory workers).[11,12] In addition, although no increase in SAB rate was observed in communities with exposure to **lead** in one study,[56] an increased risk was observed among metal workers exposed to **soldering** in radio and television manufacturing.[31]

Many cohort and case-control studies in the last decade have identified significant excess risks of SABs in various occupations in the medical profession, including **anesthesiologists,**[40] **nursing aides,**[54] **nursing assistants,**[55] and **nurses exposed to antineoplastic drugs;**[84] however some studies have observed no excess risk for laboratory workers.[2,30] A recent study of operating room staff and nurses showed a strong and significant association of exposure to antineoplastic drugs and risk of **ectopic pregnancy** (adjusted odds ratio = 10.0, 95% CL 2.1, 56.2).[77]

Finally, a few studies have focused on the risk of SAB associated with occupational **physical exertion.** Specifically, the results of a Dutch cohort study indicated that jobs involving **bending** for more than one hour per day or that produced high peak episodes of **abdominal pressure** increased SAB risk more than threefold.[19] In addition, studies in Canada[55] and in Scandinavia[63] have reported increased risks of threatened abortion or SAB associated with **standing** six or more hours per day, **working more than 40 hours per week,** or performing **heavy lifting.** Such occupational activities are potentially modifiable, and such modification of workplace activities should be undertaken for pregnant (if not all) women, even those in the early months of pregnancy.

PRETERM BIRTH

Methodologic Issues

Many of the methodologic concerns that arise in studies of occupational exposures associated with preterm birth are the same as those that arise in such studies of spontaneous abortion, discussed earlier, such as the potential for recall bias in historical cohort and case-control studies, underreporting, selection bias and misclassification of exposure. In addition, misclassification can occur in the definition of the outcome, depending on the method of its determination, i.e., weeks since last menstrual period (preterm usually is defined as fewer than 37 weeks gestation), which raises recall issues, or gestational weeks measured by ultrasound, which raises issues of observer variability and detection bias. Studies using differing definitions, such as different cutoffs of weeks of gestation to define preterm birth or detection techniques that differ in their findings, may be difficult to reconcile. Further difficulties may arise when job title is used to assess exposure and when potentially confounding variables are not controlled.[92] Finally, the role of occupation and occupational exposures in the risk of preterm birth often may be confounded by effects of social class which, in turn, may be related either to a "healthy worker effect" or an unhealthy worker effect, depending on the setting and the particular exposures being considered.[41] In general, women who work during pregnancy are healthier than those who do not,[79] which may reduce the likelihood of finding effects of employment on fetal or maternal outcomes due to the lower prevalence of risk factors (low educational level, low income, less prenatal care, smoking) for preterm birth or lower birthweight in working women.[58] Further, among working women, differences in risk factors exist across occupational sectors; for instance, operators and service workers have less education and income, late or no prenatal care, and smoke more than women in other occupations.[58,79] In addition, part-time workers are more likely to be of higher parity and to have experienced more miscarriages,[58,79] the latter increasing the risk of additional adverse pregnancy outcomes.

Occupational Exposures Related to Preterm Birth

A few studies have reported that employment outside of the home in itself is not a risk factor for preterm birth, even for manual laborers,[27] but some studies have reported an increased risk for mothers performing manual labor.[76] Just as for SAB, the increased risk of preterm birth (fewer than 37 weeks) observed in a classic French study a decade ago was observed to occur in both unskilled and clerical workers **working more than 40 hours per week** and in women working **nights** or doing **shift** work.[49] These investigators also found that the risk of preterm birth was increased in women **standing for three or more hours per day**, women involved in work requiring **physical exertion**, or women working in jobs associated with **occupational fatigue**. The relationship of the occupational risk factors to increased risk of preterm birth remained even after adjustment for high parity or nulliparity and previous premature delivery. A more recent study has also observed that gestation of fewer than 280 days was associated with physical work load, with most of the excess risk occurring in women working in agriculture and with shift work.[63] A recent large study conducted in New York examined the combined outcome of preterm (fewer than 38 weeks) and low birthweight (less than 2,500 g) in young disadvantaged white, black, and Hispanic women (ages 14–21 in 1979) and found this outcome to be related to **job-related stress** and physical exertion on the job[34] after adjusting for race, age, poverty status, education, marital status, smoking and alcohol use during pregnancy, prenatal care, pre-pregnancy weight, prior pregnancy loss, and prior low birthweight.

Studies in Canada and Scandinavia in recent years have examined the relationship of **VDT** use to course of pregnancy, and most have reported no association.[53,62] In addition, a study of **flight attendants** in Washington state reported no increased risk of prematurity (fewer than 266 days gestation) among this occupational group,[10] whose job activities expose them to a number of potential physical hazards, such as ionizing radiation, changes in circadian rhythms, long work hours, and lifting and standing for many hours.

Several studies have examined the relation of maternal occupational exposure to **metals** to preterm birth and reported a statistically significant excess risk.[76] In particular, maternal **lead** exposures have been shown to be related to risk of preterm birth. A community study conducted in the lead smelting town of Port Pirie, Australia, found a strong statistically significant relationship between preterm birth and blood lead levels at delivery (mean = 17.1 μg/L).[56] The association was dose-dependent, with a relative risk of 4.4 in mothers with the highest levels. A study using data from the federally funded U.S. National Natality and Fetal Mortality Surveys reported that maternal occupational lead exposure was associated with an increased frequency of preterm delivery (fewer than 37 weeks), as was paternal occupations in the glass, clay and stone, textile and mining industries.[78] Finally, a recent community study conducted in eastern Poland found fewer full-term births in areas with high lead and cadmium content in the soil.[43]

Several studies have examined the relationship of maternal occupation in agriculture or exposure to pesticides with adverse pregnancy outcomes other than birth defects. One California study of women attending rural health centers for a prenatal visit reported no association of maternal **agricultural work** with length of gestation or preterm delivery (fewer than 37 weeks) in this select population with access to and use of prenatal health care.[17] However, a large, nationwide study of a stratified random sample of U.S. live births reported a doubling of the risk of premature births in women working in farming, forestry and fishing.[58] A large study of women and wives of men working in the floriculture industry in Colombia reported statistically significant excesses of adverse reproductive outcomes, including prematurity (fewer than 37 weeks), during employment compared to preceding employment in this industry.[73] The authors, however, attributed most of their findings, with the exception of those pertaining to prematurity, to recall bias because (1) the unexposed jobs had the highest risk; (2) a dose-response relationship was not observed; and (3) the odds ratios were highest for employment in the more distant past, which, however, could also be due to changes in exposure over time.

One California study has reported an excess risk for prematurity (fewer than 37 weeks gestation) with self-reported occupational **solvent** exposure and a statistically significant excess (OR = 5.11, 95% CI = 1.49–17.57) for **electronic assembly** work.[48] A Scottish study also reported a statistically significant excess risk of prematurity associated with maternal, but not paternal, occupational electrical exposure and paternal, but not maternal, occupational exposure to ceramics, which may involve exposure to lead and benzene,[92] but no adjustment was made for confounding variables.[76]

BIRTHWEIGHT

Methodologic Issues

The major unique methodologic issue that arises in studies of low birthweight is that this outcome requires that a distinction be made between infants born early (preterm birth), and thus weighing less than full-term infants, and infants of low weight for their gestational age, often termed small for gestational age (SGA) or as having intrauterine growth retardation (IUGR). Preterm birth and SGA are thought to have distinct mechanisms, causes and risk factors,[41] thus emphasizing the need for their separation in epidemiologic studies. However, distinction of these outcomes requires some measure of gestational age (the preferred being ultrasound), which is often not obtained in epidemiologic studies of occupational reproductive hazards. This results in inability to distinguish these outcomes and potentially to miss detection of such exposure hazards due to the grouping of all babies with low birthweight (usually less than 2,500 g) together. Also, if gestational age is determined, different studies may measure it in different ways (maternal self-report or ultrasound), thus making this determination noncomparable in such studies. Additionally, definitions of SGA are usually based on a percentile cutoff of weight for a given gestation, but this can vary by study from the fifth[76] to the tenth[61] to quartiles,[62] thus making this outcome determination not comparable between studies. Finally, since risk factors for low birthweight differ in prevalence among working and nonworking women and among women in different sectors of the work force,[79] failure to adjust for such confounding variables can introduce bias into the results of occupational studies. In a recently published study of a large, stratified random sample of U.S. live births, Moss and Carver[58] report that after adjustment for gestational age, maternal race and age and education, marital status, parity, medical insurance, timing of prenatal care, smoking and body mass index, working during pregnancy had no effect on risk of low birthweight. One might argue that while such adjustments are essential for evaluating the effects of specific occupational chemical or physical exposures, adjustment for such variables as medical insurance and months of prenatal care may represent over-adjustments for evaluating the effect of working, since these variables are potentially informative and modifiable in the workplace.

Occupations and Exposures Associated with Low Birthweight

Nurminen and Kurppa[60] reported an adjusted risk ratio of 4.2 (95% CL 2.0, 8.7) for SGA associated with maternal exposure to occupational **noise** as assessed by industrial hygienists in nonagricultural manual workers and 4.6 (95% CL 1.3, 15.5) in manufacturing workers in Finland. The use of hearing protectors did not appear to modify this risk. Nurminen[60] also found that **shift** work was associated with a modest increase in risk of low birthweight and SGA. A study conducted in London by Rabkin and colleagues[70] found no relation of **physical effort** to birthweight, corrected for ultrasound-determined gestational age; however, Nurminen[60] reported a modest excess of SGA associated with moderate occupational physical load (adjusted risk ratio = 1.5, 95% CL 0.8, 2.8) and a higher risk in nonagricultural low-level administrative and manual workers (adjusted risk ratio = 2.4, 95% CL 1.3, 4.6) in Finland. These latter results are consistent with the findings of Homer et al.[34] showing an increased risk of low birthweight and a lower mean birthweight in young, disadvantaged women in New York who reported high levels of occupational physical exertion.

Exposure to **electromagnetic fields** has received some interest, partly due to the study in Colorado by Wertheimer and Leeper[91] showing an increased frequency of slow fetal growth when parents used electric blankets or water beds, particularly for conceptions occurring in September to June (when electric blankets would be more likely to be used and heating elements for water beds turned on), although the overall rate of slow growth as a proportion of all pregnancies did not appear to differ between users and nonusers, and no adjustment was made for confounding variables.

Nurminen and Kurppa[62] found no association of **VDT** use with birthweight in Finland. One Swedish study has reported modest elevations in risk (observed/ expected = 1.2–1.5, p < 0.05) of low birthweight in women working in jobs with moderate to high VDT use, although no accounting was made either for gestational age or confounding variables.[13] Additional studies from Montreal and California showed no significant associations of low birthweight with VDT use or trends with amount of weekly use,[53,95] although the California study did show a somewhat elevated risk of IUGR in women using VDTs greater than 20 hours per week (adjusted odds ratio = 1.6, 95% CL 0.92, 2.9) but no excess in those using VDTs fewer than 20 hours per week.

In a large study conducted in Montreal, McDonald et al.[54] found that women working in **service and manufacturing** industries had modest but statistically significant excess risks of delivering infants weighing less than 2,500 g. Sixty different industrial sectors were compared, and although care was taken to adjust for confounding variables in this study, distinction was not made between low birthweight due to preterm births and those that were SGA. In a study conducted in Scotland, Sanjose et al.[76] distinguished low birthweight from preterm birth and SGA and found increased risks of low birthweight associated with maternal work in **agricultural, electrical and leather** occupations and paternal work in **ceramics and rubber**. SGA did not appear to be related to maternal occupation, but no adjustment was made for potentially confounding variables.[92] In a study of Hispanic women seen in rural health centers in California, confounding variables were considered, and no association was found of work in agriculture with birthweight.[17] Studies of **dioxin-exposed** populations in Missouri have indicated modest, nonsignificant excesses of low birthweight and no excess of IUGR.[87]

Community studies in California on the relationship of drinking water contaminated with **organic solvents** with adverse reproductive outcomes have reported no effect,[98,99] but community studies in Michigan have reported a significant positive association of **chlorinated solvents** with risk of low birthweight.[96] In the few occupational studies that have examined the association of organic solvents to the risk of low birthweight, the results also have been conflicting. One early study showed no association with laboratory work or with occupational exposure to solvents,[2] as did a more recent study showing no excess in photolithography and diffusion workers[68] and one study showing no excess in solvent-exposed workers.[14] However, another recent study in California found a significantly increased risk in **electronic assembly** (adjusted odds ratio = 5.38, 95% CL 1.42, 20.46) and electronic production (adjusted odds ratio = 3.99, 95% CL 1.09, 14.66) workers, although no excess was observed for IUGR.[48] Further, results of analyses of the U.S. National Natality and Fetal Mortality Surveys showed a significant increased risk of SGA associated with paternal occupational exposure to benzene (odds ratio = 1.5, 95% CL 1.1, 2.3) but no relationship with maternal exposures.[78]

Regarding the relationship of **metals** to risk of low birthweight, relatively few occupational studies have been conducted. One study of Italian female lamp factory workers found no excess risk associated with **mercury**, although neither confounding nor gestational age were considered.[11] The findings from a study of Swedish dental professionals were consistent with these results.[12] A community study conducted in Australia showed no relationship of maternal blood **lead** with low birthweight or IUGR,[56] while a community study of birth in Paris did demonstrate an inverse relationship between birthweight and **cadmium** levels in the hair of newborns.[18] A Polish study also showed reduced birthweight in preterm infants born in communities with high lead and cadmium content in the soil.[43]

PREGNANCY-INDUCED HYPERTENSION

Methodologic Issues

Few studies have examined the role of occupational exposures in pregnancy-induced hypertension or preeclampsia. However, some methodologic issues unique to this set of outcomes have been raised in the few studies that have appeared. Most of these issues center around the diagnosis. Often the criteria for diagnosis are not specified, and, if they are, a distinction may not be made between cases with and without proteinuria,[50] which may denote different pathophysiologic processes.

Occupational Exposure and Pregnancy-induced Hypertension

The Finnish study of **VDTs** and adverse reproductive outcomes reported no difference in blood pressure changes over the course of pregnancy or in the occurrence of hypertension between users and nonusers.[62] However, pregnancy-induced hypertension (20 mm Hg or greater increase in mean arterial blood pressure) was associated with **shift work** in a **noisy** environment, with risk increasing with noise intensity but unrelated to the use of hearing protection.[60,61] Moderate increases in pregnancy-induced hypertension, a disorder usually arising late in pregnancy, were observed with moderate **physical work loads** in the second and third trimester, but an increasing risk with increasing load was not observed.[61] A community study from eastern Poland has reported higher mean blood pressure in pregnant women living in areas with **lead** and **cadmium** contaminated soil.[43] Finally, a strong association of preeclampsia and moderate association of hypertension with occupational **solvent** exposure has been reported in a cohort study conducted in Connecticut, but the diagnostic criteria were not available and there appeared to be no relation of outcome to duration of exposure.[14]

SUMMARY

Occupational reproductive hazards to women have been studied frequently despite the fact that many female reproductive endpoints are not readily observable or routinely recorded in occupational medical records (subfertility, delayed conception, early pregnancy loss, menstrual cycle dysfunction). However, a number of outcomes are fairly readily observable (low birthweight, clinically observed SAB, preterm labor) and medically recorded although they are not generally recorded in the occupational setting. In addition, techniques for observing reproductive outcomes in women are generally less invasive than those in men, particularly with recent developments in urinary monitoring for ovarian function and early pregnancy loss.

Although studies of some exposures and outcomes (risk of SAB, low birthweight, or preterm birth with exposure to VDTs or EMFs[13,22,38,47,53,62,65,74,81,91,95] or exposure to metals and menstrual dysfunction, infertility, or SAB[11,20,29,31,56,71]) have shown inconsistent results, a number of findings regarding other associations have been fairly consistent and are very suggestive of causal relationships. Occupational exposure to solvents does appear to increase the risk of dysmenorrhea[59,101] and SAB, particularly with exposure to organic solvents.[46,88,89,94]

Increased risk of adverse reproductive outcomes has also been observed among women working in agricultural settings, but no link has been made to specific exposures.[23,54,73] In addition, physical stressors such as shift work, long hours standing, and lifting have been fairly consistently associated with increased risk of SAB or preterm birth.[19,49,55,63] Finally, while complete agreement among studies is lacking, many have observed an increased risk of subfertility or SAB associated with work in medical occupations and with some specific medical exposures, such as nitrous oxide, anesthetic gases and antineoplastic drugs.[40,54,55,75,77,80,84]

Much remains to be explored, particularly clarification of the relationship for exposures and outcomes that have shown inconsistent results. These require specific efforts to validate exposures and outcomes, to investigate and control for confounding variables, to consider the effects of multiple comparisons, to study populations of adequate size to provide meaningful statistical analyses, and to make possible the evaluation of dose-response and timing of exposure effects.

REFERENCES

1. Ahlborg G, Hogstedt C, Bodin L, Barany S: Pregnancy outcome among working women. Scand J Work Environ Health 15:227–233, 1989.
2. Axelsson G, Lutz C, Rylander R: Exposure to solvents and outcome of pregnancy in university laboratory employees. Br J Ind Med 41:305–312, 1984.
3. Baird DD, Wilcox AJ: Cigarette smoking associated with delayed conception. JAMA 253:2979–2983, 1985.
4. Baird DD, Wilcox AJ: Effects of occupational exposures on the fertility of couples. Occup Med State Art Rev 1:361–374, 1986.
5. Baird DD, Wilcox AJ, Weinberg CR: Using time to pregnancy to study environmental exposures. Am J Epidemiol 124:470–480, 1986.
6. Baranski B: Effects of the workplace on fertility and related reproductive outcomes. Environ Health Perspect 101(suppl 2):81–90, 1993.
7. Beaumont JJ, Swan SH, Hammond SK, et al: Historical cohort investigation of spontaneous abortion in the Semiconductor Health Study: Methods and analyses of risk in fabrication overall and in fabrication work groups (unpublished manuscript).
8. Blatter BM, Zielhuis GA: Menstrual disorders due to chemical exposure among hairdressers. Occup Med 43:105–106, 1993.
9. Burch TK, Macisco JJ Jr, Parker MP: Some methodologic problems in the analysis of menstrual data. Int J Fertil 12:67–76, 1967.
10. Daniell WE, Vaughan TI, Millies BA: Pregnancy outcomes among female flight attendants. Aviat Space Environ Med 61:840–844, 1990.
11. de Rosis F, Anastasio SP, Selvaggi L, et al: Female reproductive health in two lamp factories: Effects of exposure to inorganic mercury vapour and stress factors. Br J Ind Med 42:488–494, 1985.
12. Ericson A, Kallen B: Pregnancy outcome in women working as dentists, dental assistants or dental technicians. Int Arch Occup Environ Health 61:329–333, 1989.
13. Ericson A, Kallen B: An epidemiological study of work with video screens and pregnancy outcome: I. A registry study. Am J Ind Med 9:447–457, 1986.
14. Eskenazi B, Bracken MD, Holford TR, Grady J: Exposure to organic solvents and hypertensive disorders of pregnancy. Am J Ind Med 14:177–188, 1988.
15. Eskenazi B, Gold EB, Lasley E, et al: Prospective monitoring of early fetal loss and clinical spontaneous abortion among women employed in the semiconductor industry (unpublished manuscript).
16. Eskenazi B, Gold EB, Samuels SJ, et al: Prospective assessment of the fecundability of female workers in the semiconductor industry (unpublished manuscript).
17. Fenster L, Coye MJ: Birthweight of infants born to Hispanic women employed in agriculture. Arch Environ Health 45:46–52, 1990.
18. Fréry N, Nessmann C, Girard F, et al: Environmental exposure to cadmium and human birthweight. Toxicology 79:109–118, 1993.
19. Florack EIM, Zielhuis GA, Pellegrino JEMC, Rolland R: Occupational physical activity and the occurrence of spontaneous abortion. Int J Epidemiol 22:878–884, 1993.

20. Gold EB, Eskenazi B, Hammond SK, et al: Prospectively assessed menstrual cycle characteristics in female semiconductor workers (unpublished manuscript).
21. Gold EB, Eskenazi, Lasley B, et al: Prospective methods for assessing menstrual cycle function in female semiconductor workers (unpublished manuscript).
22. Goldhaber MK, Rolen MR, Hiatt RA: The risk of miscarriage and birth defects among women who use visual display terminals during pregnancy. Am J Ind Med 13:695–706, 1988.
23. Goulet L, Theriault G: Stillbirth and chemical exposure of pregnant workers. Scand J Work Environ Health 17:25–31, 1991.
24. Gray RH, Corn M, Cohen R, et al: Final report, The Johns Hopkins University Retrospective and Prospective Studies of Reproductive Health Among IBM Employees in Semiconductor Manufacturing. May 1993.
25. Harber P: Some questions concerning "A method for monitoring the fertility of workers." J Occup Med 23:324, 1981.
26. Harlow SD, Matanoski GM: The association between weight, physical activity and stress and variation in the length of the menstrual cycle. Am J Epidemiol 133:38–49, 1991.
27. Hartikainen-Sorri A-L, Sorri M: Occupational and socio-medical factors in preterm birth. Obstet Gynecol 74:13–16, 1989.
28. Hatch M: Introduction: Biological assessments in female reproductive toxicology. Environ Health Perspect 74:55–56, 1987.
29. Heidam LZ: Spontaneous abortions among dental assistants, factory workers, painters, and gardening workers: A follow up study. J Epidemiol Community Health 38:149–155, 1984.
30. Heidam LZ: Spontaneous abortions among laboratory workers: A follow up study. J Epidemiol Community Health 38:36–41, 1984.
31. Hemminki K, Niemi M-L, Koskinen K, Vainio H: Spontaneous abortions among women employed in the metal industry in Finland. Int Arch Occup Environ Health 47:53–60, 1980.
32. Hill AB: The environment and disease: Association or causation? Proc R Soc Med 58:295, 1965.
33. Hodge HC, Smith FA: Occupational fluoride exposure. J Occup Med 19:12–39, 1977.
34. Homer CJ, James SA, Siegel E: Work-related psychosocial stress and risk of preterm, low birthweight delivery. Am J Public Health 80:173–177, 1990.
35. Howe G, Westhoff C, Vessey M, Yeates D: Effects of age, cigarette smoking and other factors on fertility: Findings in a large prospective study. BMJ 290:1697–1700, 1985.
36. Huel G, Mergler D, Bowler R: Evidence for adverse reproductive outcomes among women microelectronic assembly workers. Br J Med 47:400–404, 1990.
37. Joesoef MR, Beral V, Rolfs RT, et al: Are caffeinated beverages risk factors for delayed conception? Lancet 335:136–137, 1990.
38. Juutilainen J, Matilainen P, Saarikoski S, et al: Early pregnancy loss and exposure to 50-Hz magnetic fields. Bioelectromagnetics 14:229–236, 1993.
39. Kesner JS, Wright DM, Schrader SM, et al: Methods of monitoring menstrual function in field studies: Efficacy of methods. Reprod Toxicol 6:385–400, 1992.
40. Klebanoff MA, Shiono PH, Rhoads GG: Spontaneous and induced abortion among resident physicians. JAMA 265:2821–2825, 1991.
41. Kline J, Stein Z, Susser M: Conception to Birth: Epidemiology of Prenatal Development. New York, Oxford University Press, 1989.
42. Kuznetsova LS: The effects of the various operations in the manufacture of superphosphate on the sex organs of female workers. Gig Tr Prof Zabol 13:21–25, 1969.
43. Laudanski T, Sipowicz M, Modzelewski P, et al: Influence of high lead and cadmium soil content on human reproductive outcome. Int J Gynecol Obstet 36:309–315, 1991.
44. Lemasters GK, Pinney SM: Employment status as a confounder when assessing occupational exposures and spontaneous abortion. J Clin Epidemiol 42:975–981, 1989.
45. Levine RJ, Symons MJ, Balogh SA, et al: A method for monitoring the fertility of workers. 1. Method and pilot studies. J Occup Med 22:781–791, 1980.
46. Lindbohm M-L, Taskinen H, Sallmen M, Hemminki K: Spontaneous abortions among women exposed to organic solvents. Am J Ind Med 17:449–463, 1990.
47. Lindbohm M-L, Hietanen M, Kyyronen P, et al: Magnetic fields of video display terminals and spontaneous abortion. Am J Epidemiol 136:1041–1051, 1992.
48. Lipscomb JA, Fenster L, Wrensch M, et al: Pregnancy outcomes in women potentially exposed to occupational solvents and women working in the electronics industry. J Occup Med 33:597–604, 1991.
49. Mamelle N, Laumon B, Lazar P: Prematurity and occupational activity during pregnancy. Am J Epidemiol 119:309–322, 1984.

50. Marcoux S, Brisson J, Fabia J: The effect of cigarette smoking on the risk of preeclampsia and gestational hypertension. Am J Epidemiol 130:950–957, 1989.
51. Matsumoto S, Tamada T, Konuma S: Endocrinological analysis of environmental menstrual disorders. Int J Fertil 24:233–239, 1979.
52. McDonald AD, McDonald JC, Armstrong B, et al: Fathers' occupation and pregnancy outcome. Br J Ind Med 46:329–333, 1989.
53. McDonald AD, McDonald JC, Armstrong B, et al: Work with visual display units in pregnancy. Br J Ind Med 45:509–515, 1988.
54. McDonald AD, McDonald JC, Armstrong B, et al: Occupation and pregnancy outcome. Br J Ind Med 44:521–526, 1987.
55. McDonald AD, Armstrong B, Cherry NM, et al: Spontaneous abortion and occupation. J Occup Med 28:1232–1238, 1986.
56. McMichael AJ, Vimpani GV, Robertson EF, et al: The Port Pirie cohort study: Maternal blood lead and pregnancy outcome. J Epidemiol Community Health 40:18–25, 1986.
57. Messing K, Saurel-Cubizolles M-J, Bourgine M, Kaminski M: Menstrual cycle characteristics and work conditions of workers in poultry slaughterhouses and canneries. Scand J Work Environ Health 18:302–309, 1992.
58. Moss N, Carver K: Pregnant women at work: Sociodemographic characteristics. Am J Ind Med 23:541–557, 1993.
59. Ng TP, Foo SC, Yoong T: Menstrual function in workers exposed to toluene. Br J Ind Med 49:799–803, 1992.
60. Nurminen T: Shift work, fetal development and course of pregnancy. Scand J Work Environ Health 15:395–403, 1989.
61. Nurminen T, Kurppa K: Occupational noise exposure and course of pregnancy. Scand J Work Environ Health 15:117–124, 1989.
62. Nurminen T, Kurppa K: Office employment, work with video display terminals and course of pregnancy. Scand J Work Environ Health 14:293–298, 1988.
63. Nurminen T, Lusa S, Ilmarinen J, Kurppa K: Physical work load, fetal development and course of pregnancy. Scand J Work Environ Health 15:404–414, 1989.
64. Olsen J: Cigarette smoking, tea and coffee drinking, and subfecundity. Am J Epidemiol 133:734–739, 1991.
65. Ouellet-Hellstrom R, Stewart WF: Miscarriages among female physical therapists who report using radio- and microwave-frequency electromagnetic radiation. Am J Epidemiol 138:775–786, 1993.
66. Page H: Estimation of the prevalence and incidence of infertility in a population: A pilot study. Fertil Steril 51:571–577, 1989.
67. Panova Z, Dimitrov G: Changes in ovarian function and some functional liver indices in occupational contact with metallic mercury. Akush Ginecol (Mosk) 15:133–137, 1976.
68. Pastides H, Calabrese EJ, Hosmer DW Jr, Harris DR: Spontaneous abortion and general illness symptoms among semiconductor manufacturers. J Occup Med 30:543–551, 1988.
69. Pinney SM, Lemasters GK: A cohort study of spontaneous abortions and stillbirths in semiconductor employees. Am J Epidemiol 134:722, 1991.
70. Rabkin CS, Anderson HR, Bland JM, et al: Maternal activity and birth weight: A prospective population-based study. Am J Epidemiol 131:522–531, 1990.
71. Rachootin P, Olsen J: The risk of infertility and delayed conception associated with exposures in the Danish workplace. J Occup Med 25:394–402, 1983.
72. Rachootin P, Olsen J: Prevalence and socioeconomic correlates of subfecundity and spontaneous abortion in Denmark. Int J Epidemiol 11:245–249, 1982.
73. Restrepo M, Munoz N, Day NE, et al: Prevalence of adverse reproductive outcomes in a population occupationally exposed to pesticides in Colombia. Scand J Work Environ Health 16:232–238, 1990.
74. Roman E, Beral V, Pelerin M, Hermon C: Spontaneous abortion and work with visual display units. Br J Ind Med 49:507–512, 1992.
75. Rowland AS, Baird DD, Weinberg CR, et al: Reduced fertility among women employed as dental assistants exposed to high levels of nitrous oxide. N Engl J Med 327:993–997, 1992.
76. Sanjose S, Roman E, Beral V: Low birthweight and preterm delivery, Scotland, 1981–84: Effect of parents' occupation. Lancet 338:428–431, 1991.
77. Saurel-Cubizolles MJ, Job-Spira N, Estryn-Behar M: Ectopic pregnancy and occupational exposure to antineoplastic drugs. Lancet 341:1169–1171, 1993.
78. Savitz DA, Whelan EA, Kleckner RC: Effect of parents' occupational exposures on risk of stillbirth, preterm delivery, and small-for-gestational-age infants. Am J Epidemiol 129:1201–1218, 1989.

79. Savitz DA, Whelan EA, Rowland AS, Kleckner RC: Maternal employment and reproductive risk factors. Am J Epidemiol 132:933–945, 1990.
80. Schaumburg I, Olsen J: Time to pregnancy among Danish pharmacy assistants. Scand J Work Environ Health 15:222–226, 1989.
81. Schnorr TM, Grajewski BA, Hornung RW, et al: Video display terminals and the risk of sponaneous abortion. N Engl J Med 324:727–733, 1991.
82. [Reference deleted.]
83. Selevan SG, Lemasters GK: The dose-response fallacy in human reproductive studies of toxic exposures. J Occup Med 29:451–454, 1987.
84. Selevan SG, Lindbohm M-L, Hornung RW, Hemminki K: A study of occupational exposure to antineoplastic drugs and fetal loss in nurses. N Engl J Med 313:1173–1178, 1985.
85. Snowden R: The statistical analysis of menstrual bleeding patterns. J Biosoc Sci 9:107–120, 1977.
86. Shusterman D, Windham GC, Fenster: Employment in electronics manufacturing and risk of spontaneous abortion. J Occup Med 35:381–386, 1993.
87. Stockbauer JW, Hoffman RE, Schramm WF, Edmonds LD: Reproductive outcomes of mothers with potential exposure to 2,3,7,8-tetrachlorodibenzo-p-dioxin. Am J Epidemiol 128:410–419, 1988.
88. Swan SH, Beaumont JJ, Hammond SK, et al: Historical cohort study of spontaneous abortion in semiconductor fabrication workers: Agent level analysis (unpublished manuscript).
89. Taskinen H, Anttila A, Lindbohm M-L, et al: Spontaneous abortions and congenital malformations among the wives of men occupationally exposed to organic solvents. Scand J Work Environ Health 15:345–352, 1989.
90. Vessey MP, Wright NH, McPherson K, Wiggins P: Fertility after stopping different methods of contraception. Br Med J 1:265–267, 1978.
91. Wertheimer N, Leeper E: Possible effects of electric blankets and heated waterbeds on fetal development. Bioelectromagnetics 7:13–22, 1986.
92. Whelan E, Savitz D: Parental occupation and risk of prematurity [letter]. Lancet 338:1082, 1991.
93. Wilcox AJ, Weinberg CR, Baird DD: Caffeinated beverages and decreased fertility. Lancet 2:1453–1456, 1988.
94. Windham GC, Shusterman D, Swan S, et al: Exposure to organic solvents and adverse pregnancy outcome. Am J Ind Med 20:241–259, 1991.
95. Windham GC, Fenster L, Swan SH, Neutra R: Use of video display terminals during pregnancy and the risk of spontaneous abortion, low birthweight, or intrauterine growth retardation. Am J Ind Med 18:675–688, 1990.
96. Witowski KM, Johnson NE: Organic solvent water pollution and low birth weight in Michigan. Soc Biol 39:45–54, 1992.
97. Wong O, Morgan RW, Whorton MD: An epidemiologic surveillance program for evaluating occupational reproductive hazards. Am J Ind Med 7:295–306, 1985.
98. Wrensch M, Swan S, Lipscomb J, et al: Pregnancy outcomes in women potentially exposed to solvent-contaminated drinking water in San Jose, California. Am J Epidemiol 131:283–300, 1990.
99. Wrensch M, Swan SH, Lipscomb J, et al: Spontaneous abortions and birth defects related to tap and bottled water use, San Jose, California 1980–1984. Epidemiology 3:98–103, 1992.
100. Zhang J, Cai W, Lee DJ: Occupational hazards and pregnancy outcomes. Am J Ind Med 21:397–408, 1992.
101. Zielhuis GA, Gijsen R, van der Gulden JWJ: Menstrual disorders among dry cleaning workers [letter]. Scand J Work Environ Health 15:238, 1989.

LOWELL E. SEVER, PhD

CONGENITAL MALFORMATIONS RELATED TO OCCUPATIONAL REPRODUCTIVE HAZARDS

From the Health Risk Assessment
   Department
Battelle Pacific Northwest
   Laboratories
Seattle, Washington

Reprint requests to:
Lowell E. Sever, PhD
Battelle Seattle Research Center
P.O. Box C-5359
Seattle, WA 98105-5428

In the United States, approximately 150,000 babies are born each year with birth defects, and in 1989 birth defects were the leading cause of infant mortality in the U.S., accounting for more than 21% of all infant deaths.[7] Importantly, although the causes of some birth defects are known, approximately 60% of birth defects are of unknown etiology.[40] While exogenous agents, teratogens, account for only a small percentage of all birth defects, the recognition of the teratogenicity of drugs and chemicals has lead to concerns that occupational and environmental agents may contribute to the birth defects of unknown cause. Of particular significance is the fact that the defects that account for a large proportion of morbidity and mortality, such as neural tube defects, cardiovascular system malformations, and oral-facial clefts, are of unknown etiology.

The combination of the public health significance of birth defects, the recognition that exogenous agents can cause birth defects, the unknown etiology for most defects, and the entry of large numbers of women into occupations in which there is potential for exposure to hazardous agents has led in the last 15 years to increased concern about the relation of reproductive hazards of the workplace to risk of birth defects. There have been a number of reviews concerning this topic.[24,27,40,47,52,65] This chapter focuses on studies of birth defects published since 1988. Although developmental toxicity includes a range of endpoints, the discussion in this chapter is restricted to congenital malformations, or structural defects that have been the traditional subject of teratology. The other endpoints of interest with regard to developmental toxicity include intrauterine growth retardation, functional deficits, embryonic and fetal deaths, and childhood malignancies, the evidence for the latter two being covered in other chapters in this volume. With regard to occupational reproductive hazards, the evidence for early fetal deaths (spontaneous abortions) being associated with occupational exposures is stronger than is the evidence for congenital malformations.[23,27] Since there are biologic relationships between the developmental toxicity endpoints, and because a number of agents have been shown to cause an array of adverse outcomes, it is important to consider the possibility that an agent that is associated with spontaneous abortions may also cause congenital malformations with the appropriate timing and dose.[62]

While exposure of the conceptus to an exogenous agent is considered the usual pathway for developmental toxicity, there is also increasing evidence for male-mediated developmental toxicity.[8,44] In this review, associations between congenital malformations and both maternal/conceptus exposures and paternal exposures are considered.

For review purposes, studies of birth defects and occupational exposures have been organized in four general categories: registry-based studies, which look at parental exposure based on reported job titles or occupation and industry; pregnancy cohort studies, which consider a wide range of reported occupations; occupational cohort studies, which examine birth defect risks among workers in various occupations and with specific exposures; and case-control studies, which examine the association between cases and history of employment and/or exposure to specific chemical or physical agents in the workplace.

Exposure Assessment and Groupings

One of the key issues in occupational studies of reproductive hazards is the definition and determination of exposure. Several approaches that have been used are referred to in the discussion below. What is really of interest and concern is the dose of a specific agent that reaches either the parent's germ cells or the developing conceptus. Clearly, this level of information is unavailable, so we are left with assessment of any parental exposure to a hazardous substance. In most instances, however, we do not even have true exposure information but surrogate information such as occupation or job title. What we are usually actually dealing with, therefore, are surrogates for surrogates! Table 1 shows some of the types of exposure information used in studies of occupational reproductive hazards, listed in the order of increasing specificity.

TABLE 1.   Common Sources of Exposure Information in Studies of
Occupational Reproductive Hazards

Occupation and industry from the birth certificate
Occupation and industry from job history questionnaires
Job titles from employer records
Job-exposure matrices
Specific exposures from questionnaires
Industrial hygiene review of job titles and estimation of exposure
Specific exposures from employer records
Industrial hygiene environmental monitoring
Personal monitoring such as biomonitoring, radiation dosimetry

In a methodologic study testing the utility of the NIOSH job exposure matrix (JEM) for research on occupational teratogens, Louik and Mitchell[31] found that neither absolute attribution of exposure nor the assessment of exposure probability based on the JEM provided credible exposure measures. While it has been believed that the JEM would provide a reliable method for exposure assessment in occupational epidemiologic studies, the results described in the report of the project carried out by Louik and Mitchell are not encouraging.[31]

Of particular importance related to exposure assessment is the accuracy with which the surrogate reflects the actual exposure/dose. If there is nondifferential misclassification of exposure, any relationship between exposure and health endpoints will be biased toward no association. A common concern in studies of congenital malformations and other adverse reproductive outcomes is the possibility of biased information regarding exposure from respondents leading to differential misclassification of exposure. This has been addressed in several studies, with some authors supporting its importance[1,81] and others suggesting it may be less of a problem than commonly believed.[33]

Occupation or job title is the most frequently used surrogate for exposure. Occupations are often grouped on the basis of perceived common exposure to a specific agent or agents, for example "electrical workers" for exposure to electromagnetic fields, or a number of job titles may be combined to define "solvent exposure." Organic solvents include a extensive array of substances used widely in a number of industries for a variety of purposes, including cleaning, degreasing, extracting substances, and as chemical intermediaries. Solvents are also often components of paints, printing inks, and pesticides. Lipscomb et al. recently compiled lists of occupations that were classified as "probably solvent-exposed" and "possibly solvent-exposed."[30]

An interesting issue arises when exposures defined in this way are compared across studies and particularly across areas or countries: Are "occupations" the same in terms of potential specific exposures? If we are interested in pesticide exposure, is it logical to assume that "farmers and ranch workers" in Texas[4] are exposed to the same pesticides as "farmers and agricultural workers" in British Columbia, Canada?[45]

Another important exposure issue is the specificity of exposure within an "exposure" category. For example, solvents have been grouped by categories such as "degreasing solvents" and "nondegreasing solvents."[34] An informative example is pesticides. First, the term "pesticide" includes a wide variety of different substances that may act as fungicides, herbicides, insecticides, nematicides, and rodenticides. Secondly, organic solvents are used extensively in pesticide formulation. Thus, mixers and loaders of pesticides potentially are exposed to high levels of solvents as well as to the "active" ingredients of pesticides. For example, in a study in Italy, Petrelli et al. identified 71 different solvents in approximately 8,000 technical formulations of pesticides proposed for registration.[48]

Outcome Classification and Groupings

Questions also exist regarding the specificity and groupings of congenital malformations. It is generally believed that analyzing all "birth defects" as a group is not biologically meaningful.[64] Although most of the discussion of occupational and environmental hazards to reproduction has focused on issues of exposure, it is clear that biologically relevant classification and grouping of outcomes is also important.[62] Because of sample size and statistical power, several approaches have been taken to the grouping of defects, some of which are more logical than others. In this chapter, various combinations are described as they appear in the original literature; a full discussion of this topic is beyond this chapter's scope. This issue deserves additional attention as attempts are made to understand human developmental toxicity.

Linked Registries

A number of the studies reviewed in this chapter come from the Scandinavian countries, where high-quality registries are maintained. The use of consistent identifiers across all systems allows the linkage of workers with their spouses and with pregnancies and births. Since these countries have well-established congenital malformation registries, studies of birth defects among cohorts of workers can be carried out quite efficiently. In addition, the registries make possible large-scale case-control studies. The importance of linked registries in studies of occupational reproductive hazards has been recognized for some time,[15,58] and many of the studies reviewed illustrate this clearly.

STUDIES OF MATERNAL/CONCEPTUS EXPOSURES

Registry-based Study of Maternal Occupations

The Metropolitan Atlanta Congenital Defects Program is a population-based birth defects surveillance program in Atlanta.[14] In 1982 and 1983 an extensive interview study of cases that were identified through the registry and selected controls was carried out by the Centers for Disease Control. The primary goal was to determine whether men who had served in Vietnam were at increased risk of fathering children with birth defects.[18] A wide variety of data was collected on other potential risk factors, including parental occupations. In an article concerning these data, Erickson recently reported on 105 exposure variables and all birth defects combined (n = 4929).[16] The only significant associations with maternal employment and all birth defects were related to health care professions (health industry, OR = 1.28, 95% CI = 1.1–1.6; health occupation, OR = 1.25, 95% CI = 1.0–1.6; nurse occupation OR = 1.42, 95% CI = 1.0–2.0). These findings deserve further attention because of the wide variety of potential developmental toxicants associated with the medical environment.[40]

Pregnancy Cohort Studies of Maternal Occupations and Exposures

In the first of a series of papers based on a pregnancy cohort study in Montreal, McDonald et al. examined maternal occupations relative to the pregnancies of 56,067 women who delivered or were treated for spontaneous abortions in 11 Montreal hospitals in 1982–1984.[37] Women were identified in the hospital and were administered a questionnaire that included reproductive history, personal and social factors, and employment and personal habits during all of their pregnancies. A total of 104,649 current and previous pregnancies was ascertained. McDonald's study presents information on occupation and four adverse reproductive outcomes: spontaneous abortion, stillbirth, birthweight, and congenital defects.[37] This discussion will be restricted to congenital defects, which were grouped into a single category for these analyses.

Among women who reported their occupations as child care workers, the manufacture of metal and electrical goods, or a category of "other" service occupations, the risks for congenital defects were significantly elevated. Consistent with the association found for child care workers, an elevated but nonstatistically significantly increased risk was found among primary school teachers.

This report[37] did not explore specific exposures or defects. Evaluation of more specific defect categories and estimated exposures are considered in subsequent reports based on pregnancies from this cohort. For example, McDonald et al. examined the occurrence of congenital defects in 47,913 pregnancies among women employed for 15 hours or more per week.[36] They examined congenital defects using occupational title, chemical exposure patterns, and work requirements to define exposure. The defects were grouped into three categories: chromosomal, developmental, and musculoskeletal. The musculoskeletal defects included a variety of defects often considered to be deformations rather than malformations.[67]

Examining industrial categories, only the services sector showed a significantly increased risk of congenital defects (O/E 1.2, p = 0.02). For developmental defects (malformations) the O/E ratio was 1.14, which was significantly elevated (p = 0.02).

When 60 specific occupational groups were examined for the occurrence of defects in the above three categories, there was statistically significant heterogeneity among the chromosomal defects and developmental defects, but not for all defects combined or for musculoskeletal defects. For all defects combined, the O/E ratios were increased significantly for four occupational groups: agriculture and horticulture, telephone and postal clerks, a miscellaneous group of service occupations, and receptionists and information clerks. For the agricultural and horticultural workers the excess was mainly in the developmental defects category (O/E 4.54, p = 0.01).

When estimated exposure to chemical substances was examined, no significant associations were observed between any of the three broad defect groups and exposure to four groups of chemicals: solvents, pesticides, anesthetic gases, other chemicals.[36] Both the exposure and outcome groups were heterogeneous; statistical power to detect any biologically relevant associations would have been low because of this heterogeneity and because of the small sample size in any specific exposure or outcome group. The authors noted that two statistically significant findings deserved additional attention: eight defects, with four expected, in women who had administered antineoplastic drugs (p = 0.05) and six developmental defects observed with 1.32 expected in agriculture and horticulture workers (p = 0.01). Additional studies that address both of these issues are described below.

Occupational Cohort Studies of Maternal Exposures

Schaumburg and Olsen studied congenital malformations among births to members of the pharmacy assistants union in Denmark.[55] Pregnancies and malformations among members of this cohort were identified by linkage to the Danish Birth Registry. Exposure information was collected by questionnaire. Workers involved in the production of drugs had a statistically significantly increased risk of malformations, while the risk among those doing packaging barely failed to reach statistical significance (production, OR = 3.7, 95% CI = 1.1–12.3; packaging, OR = 4.7, 95% CI = 1.0–21.5). There was no statistically significant excess associated with exposure to any specific drug or chemical, but the adjusted odds ratio for malformations associated with solvent exposure was 2.5 (95% CI = 0.8–7.2). No information was provided on the specific malformations on which these associations were based. Solvent exposure was also significantly associated with stillbirths in this study.

Associations between both maternal and paternal exposures to anesthetic gases and congenital malformations were studied in Ontario.[21] A retrospective questionnaire-based study was carried out of 8,032 male and female operating room and recovery room personnel from 75 Ontario hospitals. Staff who were exposed to waste anesthetic gases, based on at least 2 hours per week in an operating room or recovery room, were identified. An unexposed control group of 2,525 persons working in other departments of the hospitals was identified. Past pregnancies and their outcomes were reported on the questionnaires.

The authors reported increased risks of congenital abnormalities among workers chronically exposed to anesthetic agents compared to unexposed controls.[21] For female workers, the odds ratio for congenital abnormalities associated with exposure was 2.24 (95% CI = 1.69–2.97). For male workers, the comparable odds ratio was 1.46 (95% CI = 1.04–2.05). No operational definitions of "congenital abnormalities" were given, but all anomalies were counted in the analysis and the exposed group reported a significantly higher proportion of minor malformations, such as birth marks and nevi. The authors appropriately warned that their results on congenital abnormalities must be judged with caution because of the possibility of reporting bias. The potential problems with both reporting and recall bias reflect the way the study was designed and the fact that it was a "survivor" population rather than a true historical cohort.

Skov et al. studied pregnancy outcome in a cohort of Danish nurses who handled antineoplastic drugs and a control cohort.[66] A total of 1,282 nurses from oncology departments was compared with 2,572 nurses from other departments. Pregnancy outcomes were identified by linkage to registries for spontaneous abortions and congenital malformations. Exposure was based on information provided by the head nurses from the oncology departments. There was an attempt to quantify exposure into low, intermediate, and high. No increased rates of either spontaneous abortion or congenital malformation were observed among the nurses who handled antineoplastic drugs. There were 16 malformed children among 286 children (5.59%) born to women working in the oncology departments compared to 43 malformations among 770 births (5.58%) in the comparison group. Thus, the odds ratio was 1.0. When risks were calculated based on handling antineoplastic drugs during pregnancy, the odds ratio was 1.02. The number of cases in this study was very small, and the statistical power of the study to detect an effect, if present, was low. In addition, the methods used to assess "exposure" were likely to result in a high degree of exposure misclassification.

Case-control Studies of Malformations and Maternal Occupations and Exposures

McDonald et al. carried out a nested case-control study[39] of congenital malformations identified in the Montreal pregnancy cohort study. The cohort included 56,067 women, and the case series consisted of 301 women who had a child with significant birth defect and who were employed at least 30 hours per week from conception to the end of the 12th week of pregnancy. Controls were similar in terms of employment and were individually matched to the cases on the basis of multiple factors. Occupational histories were collected by maternal questionnaires, and, for jobs in which chemical exposure was considered likely, the workplace was visited by an industrial hygienist. Attempts were made to estimate exposures to specific chemicals and severity of exposure. Two groups of defects had an excess of chemically exposed cases: cardiac defects and a category of miscellaneous defects. For cardiac defects, the matched case-control ratio was 10:5 for chemical exposures, and for miscellaneous defects, including limb deformities, the ratio was 15:7. In an analysis by nine chemical categories, only exposure to aromatic solvents showed a clear excess (OR 2.3 p = 0.04). An excess of defects, particularly of the kidney and urinary tract, was associated with exposure to aromatic solvents, especially toluene. As with many of the studies reviewed, there are potential problems with multiple comparisons of numerous exposure and outcome categories.

An array of occupations and exposures were studied in a case-control study of major malformations carried out by Cordier et al. in France.[9] The study included 325 cases of congenital malformations identified from 15 maternity hospitals and 325 controls selected from normal births occurring in the same hospitals. Occupational histories were obtained by interview, and chemical exposures and probabilities of exposures were estimated by industrial hygienists. The main occupation of interest was hospital work, and the main exposure of interest was solvents. Exposure frequencies were estimated at three levels: exposed less than 10% of work time, exposed 10–50% of work time, or exposed more than 50% of work time. Use of solvents was placed into two classes: pure solvent and products usually containing solvents. Mothers of children with oral-facial clefts were more often exposed to solvents than were mothers of the controls (OR = 7.9, 90% CI = 1.8–44.9). In addition, four of the cleft cases and none of the controls had mothers who worked as cleaners. An association betwen risk of oral-facial clefts and solvent exposure had been found in an earlier study by Holmberg and associates.[25] Cordier et al. also demonstrated associations between solvent exposure and digestive system anomalies (OR = 11.9, 90% CI = 2.0–149) and multiple anomalies (OR = 4.5, 90% CI = 1.4–16.9).[9]

No association with solvent exposure was found for central nervous system malformations in the Cordier et al. study,[9] an association that had been observed in earlier studies but not supported subsequently.[50] Roeleveld, Zielhuis, and Gabreels state that there is little evidence that structural or functional defects of the central nervous system are related to parental occupational exposure to organic solvents, but that they should be regarded as potentially hazardous to the developing brain.[50] An important consideration is the grouping of defects, since neural tube closure defects often are combined with central nervous system abnormalities with different pathogenetic mechanism. In a review of organic solvent exposure and adverse pregnancy outcomes, Taskinen interprets the literature as suggesting that maternal exposure to organic solvents during pregnancy may have adverse effects on offspring.[70] Welch also provides an excellent review of solvent exposure and pregnancy outcome.[80]

A case-control study of congenital malformations and parental employment in health care occupations was published recently by Matte, Mulinare, and Erickson.[35] The cases and controls for this study came from the Atlanta Birth Defects Case-Control Study that was described earlier.[18] Totals of 4,915 case babies and 3,027 controls was included in this analysis.

Specific birth defects were examined in 65 groups, along with all defects combined. Occupations and exposures were considered for both mothers and fathers. For maternal exposure, pregnancies were considered exposed if the woman held her job at any time from the month before through the third month after conception. For paternal exposures, jobs held 6 months before through 1 month after conception were considered. Logistic regression was used to estimate the relative risks of individual defects groups for specific groups of health care workers.

Mothers employed in an nursing occupation had a modest but statistically significant excess risk of having a child with a congenital malformation (RR = 1.42, 95% CI = 1.06–1.88). For four specific defects, the risks associated with maternal employment in nursing occupations were significantly elevated: anencephaly or spina bifida (NTDs) (RR = 2.00, 95% CI = 1.13–3.54), coarctation of the aorta (RR = 3.43, 95% CI = 1.41–8.34), genital system defects (RR = 1.61, 95% CI = 1.03–2.53), and urinary system defects (RR = 2.06, 95% CI = 1.10–3.82).

Possible exposures to the following specific agents were also evaluated: anesthetic gasses, x-irradiation, and mercury. The overall RR among mothers potentially exposed to x-irradiation was nonsignificantly elevated (RR = 2.57, 95% CI = 0.86–7.64), but there was a statistically significantly excess of NTDs (RR = 5.49, 95% CI = 1.54–25.48) based on only three cases. Potential maternal exposure to anesthetic gasses was also significantly associated with spina bifida (RR = 6.27, 95% CI = 1.20–25.03), also based on three cases. The authors discuss their findings in relation to earlier work and suggest that additional studies of maternal nursing occupations are indicated.[35] They downplay the association they found between potential for maternal x-irradiation exposure and NTDs based on a very small number of cases; this finding deserves further examination.

In a study of congenital malformations and parental occupational exposure to ionizing radiation discussed below, statistically significant associations were observed between NTDs and parental preconception radiation dose.[64] As in the Atlanta study, this was based on a small number of cases and, like Matte, Mulinare, and Erickson, these findings were not interpreted as causal.[35] Since, however, statistically significant associations were found with both paternal preconception dose ($p = 0.04$) and combined parental doses ($p = 0.02$) on the basis of tests for trend, the issue of preconception occupational radiation exposure and NTDs requires further evaluation.

A series of papers on occupational exposures and cardiovascular system malformations has been published from Finland.[74-79] There appear to be multiple publications dealing with the same cases and controls and duplication of exposure characterization. Some of the papers analyze different, but overlapping, time periods. The reports are reviewed below, the results integrated, and the overall findings interpreted.

In a 1988 paper, Tikkanen et al. published information on a series of 160 cases of cardiovascular system malformations identified from the Finnish Register of Congenital Malformations in 1980–1981 and 160 matched controls.[79] The case series excluded infants with known chromosomal anomalies. Information on parental occupations and specific exposures was obtained by maternal interview. Exposures were categorized by an industrial hygienist. There were no significant differences between cases and controls by maternal or paternal occupations. The authors reported that "the identified occupational exposures did not show any remarkable associations to cardiovascular malformations."[79]

This is apparently the only publication from the Finnish Register of Congenital Malformations that includes cases from 1980–1981. Since the study methods were similar between these cases and ones from 1982–1984 that were discussed in a number of other publications, [74-78] it is not clear why the 1980–1981 cases were not included in subsequent analyses of occupation and cardiovascular system malformations.

In a second paper, Tikkanen and Heinonen presented data on a study of cardiovascular system malformations from Finland from 1982–1984.[74] They compared 569 cases from the Finnish Register of Congenital Malformations and from the Children's Cardiac Register with 1,052 controls. Information on maternal exposures was collected by midwives using a structured interview. Exposure to organic solvents among the total case group was more prevalent than among the controls (10.4% vs. 7.8%), but this difference was not statistically significant (logistic regression adjusted OR = 1.3, 95% CI = 0.8–2.2). Exposure to organic solvents was also more prevalent among the cases of ventricular septal defect than among the controls, but again the difference was not statistically significant (OR = 1.5, 95% CI = 1.0–3.7).

In 1991, Tikkanen and Heinonen published the apparently same series of cases and controls but reported that there were 573 cases and 1,055 controls.[75] They again reported that exposure to organic solvents was slightly more prevalent among the ventricular septal defect group than among the controls (12.1% vs. 7.8%) but the difference was not statistically significant.

In 1992, Tikkanen and Heinonen published the results of a case-control study of 406 cases of cardiovascular system malformations.[70] These cases were identified from the Finnish Register of Congenital Malformations and from the Children's Cardiac Register and were born in Finland in 1982 and 1983. The control group consisted of 756 babies selected from live births without malformations during the same two years. Information on exposures to chemicals or physical factors at work was obtained by maternal interview. Maternal exposure to chemicals was significantly more prevalent in mothers of infants with cardiovascular system malformations than among mothers of controls (35.8% vs. 26.2%, $p < 0.01$).[76] Maternal exposure to dyes, lacquers, or paints also was significantly associated with risk of congenital heart defects, with ventricular septal defects and conus arteriosus syndrome showing the strongest associations. First trimester exposure to organic solvents was associated with an increased risk of ventricular septal defect ($p < 0.05$).

Tikkanen and Heinonen also published information on 50 cases of atrial septal defect from Finnish births in 1982–1983.[77] These cases were compared with 756 controls for maternal exposure to chemicals at work. Such exposure was significantly more prevalent among cases than controls (40.0% vs. 26.2%; OR = 1.9, 95% CI = 1.1–3.4). It is interesting that these same 50 cases of atrial septal defect were discussed in another paper, and the percentage of first trimester exposures in controls was different, but case and control exposures again were not significantly different, with the analysis based on chi-square tests of heterogeneity.[76]

Tikkanen and Heinonen published additional information on 90 cases of conal malformations of the heart from the 1982–1983 births.[78] Conal malformation syndrome (CAS) included anomalies such as transposition of the great vessels, Tetralogy of Fallot, and truncus arteriosus. These same 90 cases were included in an earlier paper, and the same 756 controls were used.[76] A significant association was reported between maternal exposure to dyes, lacquers, or paints at work during the first trimester and risk for CAS (OR = 2.9, 95% CI = 1.2–7.5),[77] the same finding that was reported earlier as a significant p-value, based on chi-square.[76]

In summary, the studies by Tikkanen et al. discussed above suggest potential associations between selected occupational exposures and some cardiovascular system malformations. At the same time, it is not clear why the authors examined cases from different subsets of years in different publications. The cases come from 1981–1984 and are not analyzed consistently in the reports.[74-79] This raises important questions regarding whether the reported associations would have been found if all relevant cases from the whole study period had been included in the analyses.

The Finnish findings discussed above can be compared with data reported in series of papers from the Baltimore-Washington Infant Study (BWIS) of cardiovascular system malformations. [10-12,34] The BWIS is a case-control study of cases of cardiovascular system malformations diagnosed before 1 year of age in a defined population in Maryland, the District of Columbia, and Northern Virginia. Controls are selected to be representative of the live birth cohort. Data on a variety of risk factors, including home and occupational exposures, were collected from mothers using an interviewer-administered questionnaire. Periconception exposures were defined as exposures that occurred 3 months prior to the last menstrual period through the first trimester.

In 1991 Correa-Villaseñor et al. reported on factors associated with total anomalous pulmonary venous return.[10] Studying 37 cases from the BWIS and 2,801 controls, the authors identified significant associations with maternal total lead exposure (OR = 2.93, 99% CI 1.20–7.17), painting and paint stripping (OR = 3.30, 99% CI 1.30–8.43), soldering (OR = 13.28, 99% CI 1.78–99.21), and pesticides (OR = 2.74, 99% CI = 1.17–6.44). A nonstatistically significant increased risk associated with maternal total solvent exposure was observed (OR = 3.39, 99% CI = 0.70–16.44). The authors also looked at cases of total anomalous pulmonary venus return with and without a family history of malformations. They found that the significantly increased risk associated with pesticide exposure was restricted to families with histories of both cardiac and noncardiac malformations.

Correa-Villaseñor et al. discuss their findings extensively.[10] The approach they use, a single defect category looking specifically at defects where there are and are not positive family histories, is a useful one. In their multivariate analyses, the model that best fitted the data included painting/paint stripping, soldering, pesticides, and family history. Although painting/paint stripping is included in their table under total lead exposure, the authors appropriately point out that these persons are likely to have considerable exposure to solvents. One limitation of the approach used in this study was the combination of occupational and nonoccupational exposures.

In subsequent studies from the BWIS, maternal and paternal occupations and exposures have been reported. The findings from maternal exposures are briefly summarized here and the paternal exposures later.

Magee et al.[34] examined cardiovascular system malformation risks related to maternal occupational factors in the BWIS. As noted, information regarding occupations and exposures was collected for the period 3 months prior to the estimated conception date through the first trimester. When major industrial groupings were compared between cases and controls, there were no significant differences for either mothers or fathers; because of the small numbers of parents with specific occupations, comparisons were not made at this level. The authors did, however, look at reported exposures to specific agents. Occupational and home exposures were combined and classified as positive only if narrative descriptions in the questionnaire were considered to be consistent with potential exposure.

For agents for which at least 1% of all mothers reported exposure, a significant odds ratio for all cardiovascular system malformations combined was observed only for "other solvents" (OR = 1.6, 95% CI = 1.16–2.18). The other solvents class contained nondegreasing solvents such as acetone, paint thinner, and turpentine. Two other exposures of lower frequency also showed significant (vehicular body repair work, OR = 2.34, 95% CI = 1.10–4.94) or borderline (degreasing solvents, OR = 1.73, 95% CI = 0.98–3.07) case excesses.[34]

These risks of cardiovascular system malformations associated with maternal occupational exposures reported by Magee and colleagues[34] were based on unadjusted odds ratios. Correa-Villaseñor et al.[12] expanded these analyses and presented the results of multivariate analyses. Importantly, this latter paper includes associations observed for some specific types of cardiovascular system malformations. While a thorough review of the results of these analyses is beyond the scope of this chapter, some of their findings are addressed.

One set of analyses presented unadjusted odds ratios for cases with and without genetic risk factors.[12] Interestingly, the association between cardiovascular system malformation risk and vehicular body repair work was significant only for cases with genetic risk factors, while the association with other (miscellaneous) solvents was significant only for cases without genetic factors. On multivariate analysis, both of these associations remained significant with 99% confidence intervals. Findings such as these are important in developing more specific etiologic studies.

The authors also note some of the strengths and limitations of their study with regard to understanding the possible role of a variety of factors, including occupational exposures, in the etiology of cardiovascular system malformations.[12] The study emphasizes the importance of the specificity of both outcome and exposure information. For example, relatively strong associations were observed between specific left heart defects and solvents that were diluted when all cardiovascular system malformations were analyzed as a group. Conversely, strong associations between left heart obstructions and degreasing solvents were diluted when all solvent exposure types were grouped into a single category of solvent exposure. This reflects the importance of how outcomes and exposures are defined and aggregated, as discussed in the introduction.

Different groupings of cardiovascular system malformations were used in the studies from Finland[74–79] and the BWIS.[10–12,34] The two studies show the importance of looking at individual types of defects, family history, and specific types of maternal solvent exposures in searching for etiologic clues. They also emphasize the need to consider a role for occupational/environmental agents interacting with genetic factors in the multifactorial etiology of these malformations of major public health significance.

Despite limitations in applying the NIOSH job exposure matrix to studies of birth defects, crude analysis of data from the Slone Epidemiology Unit's case-control Birth Defect Study supported associations between maternal mercury exposure and brain anomalies (based on very small numbers).[31] Consistent with the findings of McDonald et al.,[39] discussed above, they also found associations between anomalies of both the kidney and ureter and estimated exposure to the solvent benzene. Consistent with the findings of Tikkanen and Heinonen,[74] they identified significant associations between cardiovascular system malformations, specifically conotruncal defects and anomalies of the aortic valve, and xylene exposure.[31] All of these associations from the Slone Epidemiology Unit's Birth Defect Study were based on unadjusted analyses and, because of the limitations of the NIOSH JEM in assigning exposure, must be interpreted cautiously.

A number of concerns have been expressed regarding the potential developmental effects of maternal exposure to pesticides. Convincing data supporting associations between occupational pesticide exposures and congenital malformations are lacking, but several studies are highly suggestive of an effect. Some of the more recent data that contribute to this discussion are reviewed below.

Schwartz and LoGerfo conducted a case-control study of limb reduction defects identified from California birth certificates during 1982–1984.[56] They identified a total of 237 cases and selected a systematic sample of 475 live births as controls. Occupation was obtained from the birth certificate and was categorized as "agricultural" if either parent was involved in agricultural work. There was no association between parental employment in agricultural occupations and risk of limb reduction defects. Significant associations were observed between limb reduction defects and (1) maternal residence in a county with high agricultural productivity, and (2) residence in a county with high pesticide use.

It is quite likely that there is important exposure misclassification in the Schwartz and LoGerfo study. Exposure status was no more narrowly defined than that one parent worked in agriculture, and specific exposures during the sensitive period of limb development could not be determined. However, other studies suggest associations between pesticide exposure and limb reduction defects,[28,41] and this study adds to that discussion.

Restrepo et al. conducted a nested case-control study of congenital malformations in a cohort of 13,984 pregnancies among Colombian floriculture workers.[49] A total of 222 children with congenital malformations or other "congenital defects" were identified. From the same cohort, a group of 443 control births was selected and matched to the cases on maternal age and order of pregnancy. Pregnancies were defined as exposed if the mother or father had worked in floriculture during the index pregnancy. Analyses were carried out of groups of malformations and defects. The only significant association was between mother's exposure during pregnancy and birthmarks—specifically, hemangiomas, which were categorized as "congenital defects" (RR = 4.8, $p < 0.01$). The authors note that had all malformations and defects been considered together, a statistically significant association with maternal pesticide exposure would have been found ($p < 0.01$), driven entirely by the birthmark association.[49] The numbers of malformations of specific types were very limited; the leading four types of malformations that contributed to the "major malformation" group were hip dislocation, inguinal hernia, cryptorchidism, and heart murmur. The authors also note that defects leading to neonatal death "could not be assessed in the present study" and that stillbirths (late fetal deaths) were not included. No associations were found between paternal exposure to pesticides and congenital malformations or defects. It is quite likely that this study suffers from a high degree of bias in the reporting of malformations by the respondents.

A case report of malformations following maternal exposure to the insecticide oxydemoton-methyl is worth noting.[51] A farm worker, who was 4 weeks pregnant at the time of exposure, was exposed to a field contaminated with three insecticides: oxydemeton-methyl, mevinphos, and methomyl. Of these, reproductive effects have been demonstrated in test animals following exposure to oxydemeton-methyl.[51] At birth, the baby had multiple anomalies, including multiple cardiac defects, bilateral optic nerve colobomas, microphthalmia of the left eye, cerebral and cerebellar atrophy, and facial anomalies.

Zhang, Cai, and Lee conducted a case-control study of 1,013 infants with birth defects identified from 29 hospitals in Shanghai, China.[82] A matched control from the same maternity hospital was selected for each case. The mothers were interviewed to obtain information regarding occupational exposures to radiation, chemicals, pesticides and noise, and work during pregnancy. For radiation exposure prior to pregnancy, the adjusted OR was 1.9 (95% CI = 0.7–5.3), and for radiation exposure during the first trimester, the adjusted OR was 1.9 (95% CI = 0.7–4.9). Birth defects were significantly associated with exposure to chemicals before pregnancy, with an adjusted OR of 1.7 (95% CI = 1.2–2.5), and with exposure during the first trimester (adjusted OR = 3.5, 95% CI = 2.1–5.9). An association was found between central nervous system (CNS) anomalies and exposure to pesticides during the first trimester (O/E 7.5, $p < 0.01$). The CNS anomalies included ICD-9 rubrics 740–742, a pathogenetically heterogenous group of defects.

Zhang, Cai, and Lee state that their findings are consistent with previous studies and demonstrate that women exposed to pesticides had an elevated risk of birth defects.[82] In this study, however, the adjusted odds ratio for all birth defects combined and pesticide exposure during the first trimester was 1.8, but the 95% CI was 0.3–10.5. Thus, the finding of an association of all birth defects with pesticide exposure is not statistically significant. The statistically significant association between CNS anomalies and pesticides was based in three cases. Recall bias is a potential problem with this study, since information on exposure variables was obtained by maternal interview.

In a nested case-control study of congenital malformations, Taskinen, Kyyronen, and Hemminki studied pregnancies occurring in registered physiotherapists in Finland.[72] The study population included all women in the registry who had become pregnant during 1973–1982, and 46 malformation cases were identified from the Finnish Register of Congenital Malformations. Five age-matched controls were selected for each case (n = 187). Information on exposures was collected by mailed questionnaire. Deep heat therapies together and shortwaves alone were significantly associated with congenital malformations, but the increase was found only in the lower exposure category. For deep heat therapy 1–4 hours per week the OR was 2.4 (95% CI = 1.0–5.3, $p < 0.05$), and for shortwaves specifically the OR was 2.7 (95% CI = 1.2–6.1, $p < 0.05$). At the higher exposure levels—administration of the therapies five or more hours per week—there were no increases in the odds ratio. Since there were no increases at the higher exposure levels, the associations at the lower levels may not be biologically meaningful and are likely to result from recall bias. However, the risks of spontaneous abortions were elevated at the higher exposure levels, so it is possible that conceptuses with malformations due to higher exposures were more likely to be aborted spontaneously and, thus, the risk of malformations among live births is not increased. This would fit with the discussion of the "dose response fallacy" put forward by Selevan and Lemasters.[59]

Questions arose in the 1970s regarding possible associations between maternal use of video display terminals (VDTs) and adverse reproductive outcomes, particularly spontaneous abortions and birth defects. Parazzini et al.[46] recently conducted a meta-analysis of the published case-control studies. Their analyses show that the data from six studies, which examined risks of congenital malformations associated with VDTs, do not indicate increased risk. The pooled odds ratio was 1.0, with 95% CI of 0.9–1.2. No increased risk of spontaneous abortion was observed.

While most of the recent attention regarding occupational reproductive hazards has focused on exposure to specific chemical or physical agents, attention has also been paid to the effects of the physical activity associated with work on pregnancy outcome. A study by Nurminen et al. in Finland looked specifically at physical work and selected structural malformations.[42] Using a case-control design, the investigators identified 1,475 malformation cases from the Finnish Register of Congenital Malformations. The cases included 365 babies with CNS defects, 581 with oral clefts, 360 with structural skeletal defects, and 169 with cardiovascular system malformations. The controls consisted of 1,475 babies without malformations. Interviews specific to work conditions were carried out. Unexpected associations were reported between physical work load, calculated as representative energy expenditure based on work tasks, and structural malformations.[42] For CNS defects the authors reported an adjusted odds ratio of 1.7 (95% CI = 1.2–2.5) for standing work and an adjusted odds ratio of 3.0 (95% CI = 1.6–5.5) for work with moderate physical load. For oral clefts, the adjusted odds ratio was 1.8 (95% CI = 1.1–3.0), and for all defects combined it was 1.5 (95% CI = 1.1–2.0) for work with moderate physical load.

STUDIES OF PATERNAL EXPOSURE

Registry-based Studies of Paternal Occupations and Exposures

The largest study of paternal occupation and congenital malformations based on a registry population was conducted by Olshan et al.[45] This study was based on live-born cases from the British Columbia, Canada, Health Surveillance Registry. The registry is population-based and uses multiple sources to identify cases. This study was based on an analysis of children born in 1952–1973 who had birth defects in categories with a minimum of 290 cases. This resulted in 20 categories, which included a total of 14,415 cases. Two controls were selected for each case from British Columbia birth files, matched by month, year, and hospital of birth. Information regarding paternal occupation was obtained from the birth registration record. Occupation and industry were coded, and codes were grouped into 58 categories based on common work and potential exposures, as determined by an industrial hygienist.

As might be expected from a study of this size, dealing with 1,160 defect/occupation comparison, a number of statistically significant associations were found.[45] The authors are careful to point out that the study provides new leads for evaluation of the potential role of paternal occupation in the etiology of congenital malformations. The authors also provide a good discussion of the prior studies that examined some of the associations that they observed. Table 2 presents the occupation groups and defect categories for which statistically significant odds ratios were observed. With regard to specific exposures, Olshan et al. reported suggestive relationships for various defects with solvents, wood and wood products, metals, and pesticides.[45]

Prior to the above study, Olshan, Baird, and Teschke conducted a case-control study of Down syndrome and paternal occupation.[43] The study included 1,008 cases of Down syndrome, born in 1952–1973, from the British Columbia Health Surveillance Registry and two matched controls for each case. As in the study referenced aboved, paternal occupation was obtained from the birth notice. Statistically significantly elevated maternal age-adjusted odds ratios were observed for three occupational categories: janitors (OR = 3.26, 95% CI = 1.02–10.44), mechanics (OR = 3.27, 95% CI = 1.57–6.80), and farm managers/workers (OR = 2.03, 95% CI = 1.25–3.03). Exposure to hydrocarbons could be common to these

TABLE 2. Occupational Categories for Which Statistically Significant Associations Were Identified, with Defect Categories and Odds Ratios[45]

Occupational Categories	Defect	Odds Ratio	Defect	Odds Ratio	Defect	Odds Ratio
			Defect Category and Odds Ratio			
Janitors	Hydrocephalus	5.04	VSD	2.45	Other Heart	2.35
Foresters and loggers	Cataract	2.28	ASD	2.03	Syndactyly	2.03
Painters	Spina bifida	3.21	PDA	2.34	Cleft palate	3.36
Printers	Urethral atresia	4.5	Clubfoot	2.8		
Plywood mill workers	PDA	2.52	Pyloric stenosis	4.12	CDH	2.71

VSD = Ventricular septal defects
ASD = Atrial septal defects
PDA = Patent ductus arteriosus
CDH = Congenital dislocation of hip

occupations. There were several other occupations where the 95% lower limit included 1 but was > 0.9.

In a study of Prader-Willi syndrome and paternal hydrocarbon exposure cited below,[68] Down syndrome cases were selected as controls because the investigators desired controls "with a genetic disease where paternal environmental exposure was an unlikely causative factor." For evaluating paternal exposures and Down syndrome it would be important to study only trisomy cases in which the extra number 21 chromosome was paternally derived. To my knowledge this has not been done in any occupational studies, but it was in a study of parental medical x-ray exposure and Down syndrome.[69] Since approximately 80%[26] to 95%[73] of Down syndrome cases have an extra number 21 chromosome following maternal nondisjunction, paternal exposures would be irrelevant to the outcome.[61]

In the Atlanta Birth Defects Case Control Study referenced earlier, Erickson also looked at paternal occupation based on interview data.[16] For all birth defects combined, none of the odds ratios were statistically significant, i.e., the 95% CI included 1.0. The odds ratio for association of defects with paternal employment in the printing industry approached statistical significance (OR = 1.39, 95% CI = 0.9–2.2).

Pregnancy Cohort Study of Paternal Occupations and Exposures

McDonald et al. reported on paternal occupations and congenital malformations from a cohort of 56,067 pregnancies in Montreal,[38] described for maternal occupations above.[36,37,39] The interview included questions regarding father's occupation at the time of the mother's first missed menses. Occupations were classifed into six main sectors, and within those sectors 24 occupational groups were selected as having potential for harmful exposure, including probable and possible exposure to ionizing radiation. Two groups of defects were examined: (1) chromosomal defects and (2) developmental defects of the neural tube, lip and palate, heart, and of the respiratory, digestive and urinary tracts.

None of the 24 paternal occupational groups showed a statistically significant excess of chromosomal defects, and there was no heterogeneity among the 24 groups. Statistically significant heterogeneity existed for the developmental defects, and three occupational groups had statistically significant observed/ expected ratios: processing of foods and beverage, wood, and textiles; agriculture and horticulture workers; and clerical workers. For the agriculture and horticulture category, the excess was in renal and urinary tract defects. In the processing group, the excess was confined to processing of food and beverages (O/E 2.24, $p < 0.05$) but to no specific occupation within that group; excesses were observed for neural tube defects, oral clefts, digestive/respiratory defects, and renal/urinary defects. The authors note that since both the occupations and the defects observed are diverse, these findings are difficult to interpret, but the magnitude of the effects is such that they indicate the need for additional investigation.[38]

In Olshan, Teschke, and Baird's study, the odds ratio for neural tube defects among food processors was increased, but not significantly (OR = 1.20, 95% CI = 0.63–2.29).[45] A similar excess was noted for both cleft palate (OR = 1.72, 95% CI = 0.83–3.55) and cleft lip (OR = 1.42, 95% CI = 0.52–3.86), while for cleft lip plus cleft palate the odds ratio was significantly increased (OR = 2.88, 95% CI = 1.36–6.09). The concordance between the findings for food processors from these two Canadian studies indicates that this is an occupation for which additional investigation should be directed.

Occupational Cohort Studies of Paternal Exposures

Rupa et al. studied congenital defects in the offspring of 1,016 couples in India in which the fathers were occupationally exposed seasonally to a wide variety of pesticides at high concentrations in cotton fields.[53] A comparison population consisted of 1,020 couples of the same socioeconomic group and age range but without pesticide exposure. Reproductive histories were collected from the couples. A statistically significant excess of reported congenital defects in the pesticide exposed workers was observed ($p < 0.05$). The defects reported were mainly anencephaly, cleft lip and palate, club foot, limb malformations, eye deformities, and polydactyly. The reported percentage of births with malformation was 3.02% in the exposed cohort and 0.7% in the unexposed cohort. The latter number is well below the 2–3% of births usually considered to have defects observed during the newborn period, suggesting that differential reporting was a potential problem. Other studies, however, suggest associations between pesticide exposures and anencephaly,[4] cleft lip and palate,[20] limb reduction defects,[56,57] and eye defects,[13] indicating the need for further study.

Kristensen et al. studied a variety of perinatal outcomes among men in the Norwegian printing industry,[29] particularly jobs with potential for exposure to solvents and to lead. The cohort included members of four printers unions, and jobs were categorized into four exposure groups: lead only, solvents only, both lead and solvents, or "other" exposure considered not to involve solvent or lead exposure. Job category one year prior to a child's birth was used for assignment of exposure. Printers' union records were linked to the Medical Birth Registry of Norway, identifying 6,251 infants born to members during 1967–1986. All births occurring in Oslo during the same period were used as an external control population.

Although increased risks of selected birth defects among children of printers have been observed in some studies,[17,45] this study failed to demonstrate such increased risks, as the standarized morbidity ratio (SMR) for all defects was 0.9 (95% CI = 0.78–1.0). The SMR for cleft lip and palate was 1.6, which approached statistical significance (95% CI = 0.97–2.5). A clustering of cleft lip was observed in the two categories of paternal lead exposures, mainly among boys. The increased SMR for boys with fathers in those two categories was statistically significant (SMR = 4.1, 95% CI = 1.8–8.1). No increased malformation risks were observed among the offspring of men with solvent exposure.

An association between paternal employment in the printing industry and cleft palate had been demonstrated earlier by Erickson, Cochran, and Anderson.[17] In Olshan, Teschke, and Baird's study, the defects associated with printing are shown in Table 2.[45] The odds ratio for cleft palate was 1.55 (95% CI = 0.34–7.10), for cleft lip 1.0 (95% CI = 0.09–11.06), and for cleft lip plus cleft palate 1.15 (95% CI = 0.29–4.52). While there was no specific consideration of lead, the authors did note that exposure to metals was common to a number of occupations associated with increased birth defect risks, including cleft palate.[45] No associations of printing with birth defects was observed, however, in McDonald's study of paternal exposures.[38]

Bonde, Olsen, and Hansen, with a particular interest in exposure to welding, examined a variety of adverse pregnancy outcomes in a Danish cohort of metal workers.[3] A total of 3,569 children, born to 8,376 men who completed a mailed exposure questionnaire, was identified from the Medical Birth Register of Denmark for the period 1973–1986. There was no evidence of increased risks of congenital malformations associated with welding. There was, in fact, a significantly reduced risk among children whose fathers were exposed to mild steel welding only (OR = 0.57, 95% CI = 0.41–0.80). The authors hypothesize that since reduced fertility has been reported among mild steel welders,[2] conceptions occurring in spite of mild steel exposure are at decreased risk of developing congenital malformations. This is highly speculative, and a mechanism for this hypothesis is not readily apparent. In Olshan, Teschke, and Baird's study, discussed earlier, no association, positive or negative, was observed between congenital malformations and welding.[45]

Case-control Studies of Malformations and Paternal Occupations and Exposures

Sever et al. examined the association between parental occupational exposure to ionizing radiation and congenital malformations.[64] Cases of congenital malformations occurring from 1957 through 1980 were identified in the two counties in the vicinity of the Hanford Nuclear Facility in southeastern Washington state, where the Hanford site has been a major employer. A total of 672 cases were identified using multiple sources, and 977 matched controls were selected based on birth certificates and hospital birth records. Parents of cases and controls were linked to employment rosters of employees at the Hanford site. For parents who were employed there, data were obtained on occupational radiation exposure of both parents prior to conception and for mothers' exposure during gestation. Based on job title information from the birth certificate and from employment records, information also was obtained on potential for exposure to other harmful substances.

Twelve specific malformation categories, as well as major malformations and all malformations as a group, were analyzed for association with Hanford employment and with occupational radiation dose. Two defects, tracheoesophageal fistula and congenital dislocation of the hip, were significantly associated with paternal Hanford employment but not with radiation exposure. Neural tube defects showed a significant association with paternal radiation dose, on the basis of a one-tailed test for trend ($p = 0.04$). When combined maternal and paternal doses were considered, the association between dose and neural tube defect risk remained statistically ($p = 0.02$). No significant associations were found for Down syndrome, for which an association with radiation was considered most likely a priori.[64] When all malformations were considered as a group, the relationship to both paternal and combined parental radiation exposure before conception was in the positive direction ($0.05 < p < 0.10$). Examination of specific job categories and potential chemical exposures did not show any associations with neural tube defects.

While the association between neural tube defects and paternal occupational radiation exposure was not considered by the authors to be causal, the recent identification of a similar association between paternal radiation and risk of childhood leukemia, discussed in chapter 10, indicates the need for further consideration of this issue. Since the number of mothers who had gestational exposures to ionizing radiation was very small, this study does not contribute to our understanding of the teratogenicity of in utero radiation exposure, which is known to be harmful to the developing central nervous system.[61]

An interesting finding in the past few years relevant to paternal exposures and birth defects is the reported association of Prader-Willi syndrome with paternal exposure to hydrocarbons. Prader-Willi syndrome is a multiple-anomaly disorder characterized by hypotonia, obesity, hypogonadism, short stature, mental deficiency, and other phenotypic features.[5] In 1987 Strakowski and Butler carried out a case-control study of paternal occupations and Prader-Willi syndrome.[68] Controls were children with Down syndrome or fragile X syndrome. Paternal occupations were grouped into categories that had potential for hydrocarbon exposure, potential for lead exposure, potential for both, or potential for neither. Strakowski and Butler observed a significantly increased proportion of occupations with potential for hydrocarbon exposure among the Prader-Willi syndrome cases compared with the controls (20.8% vs. 12.0%, $p < 0.001$).[68] No association was observed with lead exposure.

In approximately 50–70% of Prader-Willi syndrome cases there is a de novo interstitial deletion in chromosome 15.[6] Studies of chromosome polymorphisms show that the deletion occurs most commonly in the paternally derived chromosome. In the Strakowski and Butler series, 24% of the cases with a recognizable deletion had a father with occupational hydrocarbon exposure.[68] In a later series reported by Cassidy, Gainey, and Butler, the paternal occupations of 81 individuals with Prader-Willi syndrome were studied, 53 cases with recognizable deletions and 28 cases without.[6] Of the cases with deletions, 45% of the fathers were employed in hydrocarbon-exposed occupations, as were 54% of the nondeletion cases. This supports the suggestion of a relationship between paternal hydrocarbon exposure and Prader-Willi syndrome. It also supports suggestions that microdeletions on chromosome 15 may be involved in cases of Prader-Willi syndrome in which no recognizable deletion is found.[5,6]

In this author's opinion, the suggestion of an association between paternal hydrocarbon exposure and Prader-Willi syndrome, related to a chromosomal deletion, is particularly interesting. It provides a mechanism through which male-mediated developmental effects could occur. It is also of particular relevance to some of the possible contributions of the technology growing out of the Human Genome Project and our understanding of the etiology of birth defects. It supports parallels between the etiology of childhood cancers and some birth defects, as paternal hydrocarbon exposure has also been suggested to be associated with childhood cancers.[19] In addition, some solvents are hydrocarbons, and, as discussed, both maternal and paternal solvent exposure has been associated with several congenital malformations for which the etiology is otherwise unknown.

Taskinen et al. conducted a nested case-control study of congenital malformations in a cohort of Finnish men who were biologically monitored for exposure to six organic solvents.[71] The men's wives were identified through a population register, and pregnancies were identified through the Hospital Discharge Register. Congenital malformations occurring among births to this cohort during 1973–1982 were identified from the Finnish Register of Congenital Malformations. The exposure of the men during the spermatogenesis cycle preceding the pregnancies and the exposure of the women during the first trimester were determined by questionnaire. Exposure assessment was based on occupation, job description, reported solvent or other chemical usage, and biological monitoring data. The likelihood of exposure during the 80 days prior to conception was determined. The odds ratio for spontaneous abortions was significantly elevated (OR = 2.39, 95% CI = 1.1–5.0). There was no association between paternal solvent exposure and congenital malformations, but the total number of cases was small—25, seven of which were congenital dislocations of the hip—so the statistical power was extremely limited.

Brender and Suarez carried out a case-control study of anencephaly in Texas.[4] Cases were identified from vital records for 1981–1986 and were compared to a series of controls selected from live births during the same period and frequency matched to the cases by race, ethnicity, and year of birth. Parental occupations were obtained from the vital records, and occupations with potential for exposure to pesticides and solvents were identified. For the group of paternal occupations associated with solvent exposure, there was a significantly increased odds ratio (OR = 2.53, 95% CI = 1.56–4.10). For painters, the odds ratio was 3.43 (95% CI = 1.83–6.43). In a review, Taskinen noted that paternal exposure to organic solvents before conception may have adverse effects on pregnancy and offspring.[70] As mentioned above, maternal solvent exposure has been suggested to be associated with a variety of malformations but not supported by the Taskinen study reviewed above.[71]

Brender and Suarez also examined the association between anencephaly and paternal pesticide exposure.[4] For the group of paternal occupations with estimated exposure to pesticides, the odds ratio was 1.28, which was not statistically significantly elevated (95% CI = 0.77–2.13). For farmers and ranch workers, the odds ratio was 1.73, again an increase which was not statistically significant (95% CI = 0.84–3.55). Brender and Suarez[4] review some of the studies that suggest possible associations between neural tube defects, including anencephaly, and pesticide exposure. I share their assessment that additional studies need to be carried out examining this possible association. As noted earlier, the use of solvents in pesticide formulations and the suggestions of associations between both solvent and pesticide exposure and neural tube defects increases the importance of such studies, particularly in areas where rates of neural tube defect are high.

In the report from the Slone Epidemiology Unit referenced above, Louik and Mitchell reported significant associations between CNS malformations, specifically anencephaly and hydrocephaly/ventriculomegaly, and paternal mercury exposure.[31] These findings were based on a small number of cases. Of greater interest is the fact that they also observed increased risks of neural tube defects associated with paternal solvent exposure. For spina bifida there was a statistically significant association with xylene, and for anencephaly and spina bifida there was a statistically significant association with benzene. These findings, contained in an unpublished report to NIOSH,[31] are consistent with the associations observed between paternal solvent exposure and anencephaly reported by Brender and Suarez[4] and, similarly, with the association between paternal employment as a painter and spina bifida.[45] However, as noted earlier in the analysis of maternal exposures, the findings from the Slone Epidemiology Unit are based on unadjusted odds ratios, and the accuracy of the exposures assigned on the basis of the NIOSH JEM is highly questionable.

In addition to the maternal exposures discussed earlier, the investigators for the BWIS studied cardiovascular system malformations and paternal exposures.[11] Based on a small number of exposed cases, risks of atrial septal defect and of membranous ventricular septal defect were significantly elevated among fathers exposed to jewelry making. Cases of pulmonary atresia and of endocardial cushion defect with Down syndrome had elevated odds of paternal exposure to lead soldering and welding, respectively. Information on the specific type of welding was not provided. Cases of endocardial cushion defect without Down syndrome showed an unadjusted odds ratio fo 5.1 for paternal exposure to ionizing radiation. Interestingly, when the odds ratio was adjusted to control for potential confounders it was reduced to 1.8 due to a strong correlation between paternal exposure to ionizing radiation and the presence of a genetic disorder in the subject. This finding certainly deserves further evaluation. Additional analyses and the importance of considering family history, genetic disorders, and the presence of the father at the interview are discussed in this report.[11]

Paternal exposures in the BWIS study were also reported on by Magee et al. for all cardiovascular system malformations combined.[34] The only paternal chemical exposure that showed a statistically significant association was "other solvents" (OR = 1.26, 95% CI = 1.06–1.49). No associations were observed between case and control fathers and individual occupational or industrial groups. An unanticipated finding reported by Magee et al. was an association between cardiovascular system malformation risk and paternal industrial exposure to extreme cold (OR = 2.24, 95% CI = 1.01–4.96).[34] To my knowledge, no other studies of congenital malformations and paternal cold exposure have been reported.

Lead has been recognized for many years as a reproductive and developmental toxicant.[63] Hakim and associates reported a weak association between paternal occupational lead exposure and strabismus in a case-control study.[22] Although the authors state "the study results suggest the possibility of a weak association," the unadjusted findings were as follows for the esotropic form of strabismus: low exposure (OR = 1.0, 95% CI = 0.5–2.1), moderate exposure level (OR = 2.1, 95% CI = 0.9–5.3) and high exposure (OR = 1.2, 95% CI = 0.4–3.3). It is difficult to interpret these findings as being of biological significance.

Sallmén et al. conducted a nested case-control study of congenital malformations in a cohort of men working in a variety of industries in Finland who were biologically monitored for lead exposure.[54] The cohort was identified from records of the Institute of Occupational Health; their wives were identified from the Finnish Central Population Registry; pregnancies (births) during 1973–1982 were identified from the nationwide database on medically diagnosed pregnancies; and malformation cases were ascertained from the Finnish Register of Congenital Malformations. From a total of 51 malformation cases identified, 27 who met combined requirements of responding to a mailed questionnaire and having what were considered to be reliable estimates of exposure proximate to the pregnancy were included. Three controls were selected for each case (n = 57).

Among the fathers of cases, 10 (37%) had blood lead levels that exceeded 1.0 μmol/L, compared to 11 controls (19%). The odds ratio for congenital malformations associated with lead exposure was 2.4, which did not reach statistical significance (95% CI 0.9–6.5). The malformations included were heterogeneous, and the statistical power of this study is low. The findings were interpreted as providing limited support for the hypothesis that paternal lead exposure is associated with congenital malformations.

CONCLUSION

In a recent review article on occupational exposures and reproduction, Hatch and Marcus state: "Congenital malformations, either in miscarriages or at birth, have not yet been convincingly shown to be related to occupational exposures in women."[23] I believe this remains true. At the same time, evidence is increasing that concerns about this issue, and paternal exposures as well, are not misplaced. The key word here is "convincingly."

The studies reviewed in this chapter suggest that for a number of the more common congenital malformations of unknown etiology there may be associations with workplace exposures of either parent, particularly solvents and pesticides. This includes neural tube defects, cleft lip and palate, and some cardiovascular system malformations.

Important issues involve the adequacy of studies to evaluate potential risks. Case-control studies of individual types of malformations are often limited by small sample size and the relative infrequency of specific exposures. Cohort studies are limited by the low prevalence at birth of even the most common malformations. Complicating both case-control and cohort studies are major issues related to the accuracy and specificity of assessment/classification of exposure, let alone dose, classification and grouping of malformations, and multiple comparisons. We address some of the major concerns regarding exposure assessment and dose in chapter 10, and those points are also applicable here.

There are a number of advantages to the methods of study possible in the Scandinavian countries, where information on individuals can be linked from a variety of data sources. The use of large population-based registries such as the Metropolitan Atlanta Congenital Defects Program and the British Columbia Health Surveillance Registry for generating hypotheses is important.

To develop a better understanding of potential associations between congenital malformations and occupational exposures requires a collaborative multicenter approach along with a refinement of exposure characterization. The potential role of biomarkers in studying occupational exposures and congenital malformations needs to be considered more extensively.[32] New approaches to the grouping of malformations on the basis of shared pathogenesis need to be explored. Finally, it is likely that with the expansion of our ability to study genetic material—a result of the Human Genome Project—new techniques will be provided for studying human congenital malformations associated with occupational exposures. The example of paternal hydrocarbon exposures associated with chromosomal microdeletions leading to Prader-Willi syndrome discussed above provides a possible prototype of such phenomena.

REFERENCES

1. Ahlborg GA Jr: Validity of exposure data obtained by questionnaire: Two examples from occupational reproductive studies. Scand J Work Environ Health 16:284–288, 1990.

2. Bonde JP, Hanson SK, Levine RD: Fertility among Danish male welders. Scand J Work Environ Health 16:315–322, 1990.
3. Bonde JPE, Olsen JH, Hansen KS: Adverse pregnancy outcome and chilhood malignancy with reference to paternal welding exposure. Scand J Work Environ Health 18:169–177, 1992.
4. Brender JD, Suarez L: Paternal occupation and anencephaly. Am J Epidemiol 131:517–521, 1990.
5. Butler MG: Prader-Willi Syndrome: Current understanding of cause and diagnosis. Am J Med Genet 35:319–332, 1990.
6. Cassidy SB, Gainey AJ, Butler MG: Occupational hydrocarbon exposure among fathers of Prader-Willi Syndrome patients with and without deletions of 15q. Am J Hum Genet 44:806–810, 1989.
7. Centers for Disease Control: Current trends: Infant mortality-United States, 1990. MMWR 42:161–165, 1993.
8. Colie CF: Male-mediated teratogenesis. Reprod Toxicol 7:3–9, 1991.
9. Cordier S, Ha M-C, Ayme S, Gouhard J: Maternal occupational exposure and congenital malformations. Scand J Work Environ Health 18:11–17, 1992.
10. Correa-Villaseñor A, Ferencz C, Boughman JA, Neill CA (Baltimore-Washington Infant Study Group): Total anomalous pulmonary venous return: Familial and environmental factors. Teratology 44:415–428, 1991.
11. Correa-Villaseñor A, Ferencz C, Loffredo C, Magee C: Paternal exposures and cardiovascular malformations. J Exp Anal Environ Epidemiol 3:173–185, 1993.
12. Correa-Villaseñor A, Wilson PD, Loffredo CA, et al: Risk factor analysis. In Ferencz C, Rubin JD, Loffredo CA, Magee CA (eds): Perspectives in Pediatric Cardiology, Vol 4. New York, Futura Publishing, 1993, pp 233–247.
13. Dolk H, Elliott P: Evidence for "clusters of anophthalmia" is thin. BMJ 307:203, 1993.
14. Edmonds LD, Layde PM, James LM, et al: Congenital malformations and surveillance: Two American systems. Int J Epidemiol 10:247–252, 1981.
15. Erickson JD: Assessing occupational hazards to reproduction: Uses of existing data sets. In Lockey JE, Lemasters GK, Keye WR Jr (eds): Reproduction: The New Frontier in Occupational and Environmental Health Research. Prog Clin Biol Res 160:99–107, 1984.
16. Erickson JD: Risk factors for birth defects: Data from the Atlanta Birth Defects Case-Control Study. Teratology 43:41–51, 1991.
17. Erickson JD, Cochran WM, Anderson CE: Parental occupation and birth defects: A preliminary report. Contrib Epidemiol Biostat 1:107–117, 1979.
18. Erickson JD, Mulinare J, McClain PW, et al: Vietnam veterans' risks for fathering babies with birth defects. JAMA 252:903–912, 1984.
19. Gold EB, Sever LE: Childhood cancers associated with parental occupational exposures. Occup Med State Art Rev 9:495–539, 1994.
20. Gordon JE, Shy CM: Agricultural chemical use and congenital cleft lip and/or palate. Arch Environ Health 36:213–220, 1981.
21. Guirguis SS, Pelmear PL, Roy ML, Wong L: Health effects associated with exposure to anaesthetic gases in Ontario hospital personnel. Br J Ind Med 47:490–497, 1990.
22. Hakim RB, Stewart WF, Canner JK, Tielsch JM: Occupational lead exposure and strabismus in offspring: A case-control study. Am J Epidemiol 133:351–356, 1991.
23. Hatch M, Marcus M: Occupational exposures and reproduction. In Kiely M (ed): Reproductive and Perinatal Epidemiology. Boca Raton, CRC Press, 1991, pp 131–142.
24. Hatch M, Stein ZA: Agents in the workplace and effects on reproduction. Occup Med 1:531–534, 1986.
25. Holmberg PC, Hernberg S, Kurppa K, et al: Oral clefts and organic solvent exposure during pregnancy. Int Arch Occup Environ Health 50:371–376, 1982.
26. Juberg RC, Mowrey PN: Origin of nondisjunction of Trisomy 21 Syndrome: All studies compiled, parental age analysis, and international comparisons. Am J Med Genet 16:111–116, 1983.
27. Kline JK: Maternal occupation: Effects on spontaneous abortion and malformations. Occup Med 1:381–403, 1986.
28. Kricker A, McCredie J, Elliott J, Forrest J: Women and the environment: A study of congenital limb anomalies. Comm Health Stud 10:1–11, 1986.
29. Kristensen P, Irgens LM, Dalveit AK, Andersen A: Perinatal outcome among children of men exposed to lead and organic solvents in the printing industry. Am J Epidemiol 137:134–144, 1993.
30. Lipscomb JA, Fenster L, Wrensch M, et al: Pregnancy outcomes in women potentially exposed to occupational solvents and women working in the electronics industry. J Occup Med 33:597–604, 1991.

31. Louik C, Mitchell AA: Occupational Exposures and Birth Defects: Final performance report. Grant 1RO1OH02598-O1A1. National Institute for Occupational Safety and Health, May 28, 1992.
32. Lynberg MC, Khoury MJ: Interaction between epidemiology and laboratory sciences in searching for causes of birth defects in humans. J Toxicol Environ Health 40:435–444, 1993.
33. MacKenzie SG, Lippman A: An investigation of report bias in a case-control study of pregnancy outcome. Am J Epidemiol 129:65–75, 1989.
34. Magee CA, Loffredo CA, Correa-Villaseñor A, Wilson PD: Environmental factors in occupations, home, and hobbies. In Ferencz C, Rubin JD, Loffredo CA, Magee CA (eds): Perspectives in Pediatric Cardiology, Vol 4. New York, Futura Publishing, 1993, pp 207–231.
35. Matte TD, Mulinare J, Erickson JD: Case-control study of congenital defects and parental employment in health care. Am J Ind Med 24:11–23, 1993.
36. McDonald AD, McDonald JC, Armstrong B, et al: Congenital defects and work in pregnancy. Br J Ind Med 45:581–588, 1988.
37. McDonald AD, McDonald JC, Armstrong B, et al: Occupation and pregnancy outcome. Br J Ind Med 44:521–526, 1987.
38. McDonald AD, McDonald JC, Armstrong B, et al: Fathers' occupation and pregnancy outcome. Br J Ind Med 46:329–333, 1989.
39. McDonald JC, LaVoie J, Coté R, McDonald AD: Chemical exposures at work in early pregnancy and congenital defect: A case-referent study. Br J Ind Med 44:527–533, 1987.
40. Mortensen ML, Sever LE, Oakley GP Jr: Teratology and the epidemiology of birth defects. In Gabbe SG, Niebyl JR, Simpson JL (eds): Obstetrics: Normal and Problem Pregnancies. 2nd ed. New York, Churchill Livingstone, 1991, pp 233–268.
41. Munger R, Isacson P, Kramer M, et al: Birth defects and pesticide-contaminated water supplies in Iowa. Am J Epidemiol 136:959, 1992.
42. Nurminen T, Lusa S, Ilmarinen J, Kurppa K: Physical work load, fetal development and course of pregnancy. Scand J Work Environ Health 15:404–414, 1989.
43. Olshan AF, Baird PA, Teschke K: Paternal occupational exposures and the risk of Down syndrome. AM J Hum Genet 44:646–651, 1989.
44. Olshan AF, Faustman EM: Male-mediated developmental toxicity. Reprod Toxicol 7:191–202, 1993.
45. Olshan AF, Teschke K, Baird PA: Paternal occupation and congenital anomalies in offspring. Am J Ind Med 20:447–475, 1991.
46. Parazzini F, Luchini L, La Vecchia C, Crosignani PG: Video display terminal use during pregnancy and reproductive outcome—a meta-analysis. J Epidemiol Commun Health 47:265–268, 1993.
47. Paul M (ed): Occupational and Environmental Reproductive Hazards: A Guide for Clinicians. Baltimore, Williams & Wilkins, 1992.
48. Petrelli G, Siepi G, Miligi L, Vineis P: Solvents in pesticides. Scand J Work Environ Health 19:63–65, 1993.
49. Restrepo M, Muñoz N, Day N, et al: Birth defects among children born to a population occupationally exposed to pesticides in Colombia. Scand J Work Environ Health 16:239–246, 1990.
50. Roeleveld N, Zielhuis GA, Gabreels F: Occupational exposure and defects of the central nervous system in offspring: Review. Br J Ind Med 47:580–588, 1990.
51. Romero P, Barnett PG, Midtling JE: Congenital anomalies associated with maternal exposure to oxydemeton-methyl. Environ Res 50:256–261, 1989.
52. Rosenberg MJ, Feldblum PJ, Marshall EG: Occupational influences on reproduction: A review of recent literature. J Occup Med 29:584–591, 1987.
53. Rupa DS, Reddy PP, Reddi OS: Reproductive performance in population exposed to pesticides in cotton fields in India. Environ Res 55:123–128, 1991.
54. Sallmén M, Lindbohm M-L, Anttila A, et al: Paternal occupational lead exposure and congenital malformations. J Epidemiol Community Health 46:519–522, 1992.
55. Schaumburg I, Olsen J: Congenital malformations and death among the offspring of Danish pharmacy assistants. Am J Ind Med 18:555–564, 1990.
56. Schwartz DA, LoGerfo JP: Congenital limb reduction defects in the agricultural setting. Am J Public Health 78:654–659, 1988.
57. Schwartz DA, Newsum LA, Heifez RM: Parental occupation and birth outcome in an agricultural community. Scand J Work Environ Health 12:51–54, 1986.
58. Selevan SG, Hemminki K, Lindbohm M-L: Linking data to study reproductive effects of occupational exposures. Occup Med 1:445–455, 1986.
59. Selevan SG, Lemasters GK: The dose-response fallacy in human reproductive studies of toxic exposures. J Occup Med 29:451–454, 1987.

60. Sever LE: Neuroepidemiology of intrauterine radiation exposure. In Molgaard CA (ed): Neuroepidemiology: Theory and Method. Orlando, Academic, 1992, pp 241–256.
61. Sever LE: Parental radiation exposure and children's health: Are there effects on the second generation? Occup Med 6:613–627, 1991.
62. Sever LE: The state of the art and current issues regarding reproductive outcomes potentially associated with environmental exposures: Reduced fertility, reproductive wastage, congenital malformations, and birth weight. Work Group on Reproductive and Developmental Epidemiology: Research Issues. Cincinnati, October 24–26, 1988, US Enviromental Protection Agency report 600/8–89/103.
63. Sever LE, Hessol NA: Toxic effects of occupational and environmental chemicals on the testes. In Thomas JA, Korach KS, McLachlan JA (eds): Endocrine Toxicology. New York, Raven, 1985, pp 211–248.
64. Sever LE, Gilbert ES, Hessol NA, McIntyre JM: A case-control study of congenital malformations and occupational exposure to low-level radiation. Am J Epidemiol 127:226–242, 1988.
65. Shaw GM, Gold EB: Methodological considerations in the study of parental occupational exposures and congenital malformations in offspring. Scand J Work Environ Health 14:344–355, 1988.
66. Skov T, Maarup B, Olsen J, et al: Leukaemia and reproductive outcome among nurses handling antineoplastic drugs. Br J Ind Med 49:855–861, 1992.
67. Smith DW: Recognizable Patterns of Human Malformation: Genetic, Embryonic and Clinical Aspects. 2nd ed. Philadelphia, WB Saunders, 1976.
68. Strakowski SM, Butler MG: Paternal hydrocarbon exposure in Prader-Willi syndrome. Lancet 2:1458, 1987.
69. Strigini P, Pierluigi M, Forni GL, et al: Effect of x-rays on chromosome 21 nondisjunction. Am J Med Genet Suppl 7:155–159, 1990.
70. Taskinen HK: Effects of parental occupational exposures on spontaneous abortion and congenital malformation. Scand J Work Environ Health 16:297–314, 1990.
71. Taskinen H, Anttila A, Lindbohm M-L, et al: Spontaneous abortions and congenital malformations among the wives of men occupationally exposed to organic solvents. Scand J Work Environ Health 15:345–352, 1989.
72. Taskinen H, Kyronen P, Hemminki K: Effects of ultrasound, shortwaves, and physical exertion on pregnancy outcome in physiotherapists. J Epidemiol Comm Health 44:196–201, 1990.
73. Thompson M, McInnis R, Willard H: Genetics in Medicine. 5th ed. Philadelphia, WB Saunders, 1991.
74. Tikkanen J, Heinonen OP: Cardiovascular malformations and organic solvent exposure during pregnancy in Finland. Am J Ind Med 13:1–8, 1988.
75. Tikkanen J, Heinonen OP: Maternal exposure to chemical and physical factors during pregnancy and cardiovascular malformations in the offspring. Teratology 43:591–600, 1991.
76. Tikkanen J, Heinonen OP: Occupational risk factors for congenital heart disease. Int Arch Occup Environ Health 64:59–64, 1992.
77. Tikkanen J, Heinonen OP: Risk factors for atrial septal defect. Eur J Epidemiol 8:509–515, 1992.
78. Tikkanen J, Heinonen OP: Risk factors for conal malformations of the heart. Eur J Epidemiol 8:48–57, 1992.
79. Tikkanen J, Kurppa K, Timonen H, et al: Cardiovascular malformations, work attendance, and occupational exposures during pregnancy in Finland. Am J Ind Med 14:197–204, 1988.
80. Welch LS: Organic solvents. In Paul M (ed): Occupational and Environmental Reproductive Hazards: A Guide for Clinicians. Baltimore, Williams & Wilkins, 1993, pp 267–279.
81. Werler MM, Pober BR, Nelson K, Holmes LB: Reporting accuracy among mothers of malformed and nonmalformed infants. Am J Epidemiol 129:415–421, 1989.
82. Zhang J, Cai W-W, Lee DJ: Occupational hazards and pregnancy outcomes. Am J Ind Med 21:397–408, 1992.

ELLEN B. GOLD, PhD
LOWELL E. SEVER, PhD

CHILDHOOD CANCERS ASSOCIATED WITH PARENTAL OCCUPATIONAL EXPOSURES

From the Health Risk Assessment
Department
Battelle Pacific Northwest
Laboratories
Seattle, Washington (LES)
and
Division of Occupational/
Environmental Medicine and
Epidemiology
School of Medicine and Institute
of Toxicology and
Environmental Health
University of California
Davis, California (EBG)

Reprint requests to:
Ellen B. Gold, PhD
Associate Professor
Division of Occupational/
Environmental Medicine
and Epidemiology
Institute of Toxicology
and Environmental Health
University of California
Davis, CA 95616-8648

Supported by a Research Career
Development Award from the Na-
tional Institute of Environmental
Health Sciences, 5 K04 ES00202-4
(EBG).

The incidence of cancer in children younger than 15 has been increasing over the past two decades in the United States, with white children in this age group showing an incidence of 12.7 per 100,000 in 1973 and 14.1 in 1988 (r = 0.542, p = 0.03).[1] In particular, the increases over this time have been largest among the three most frequent types of childhood cancer: acute lymphocytic leukemia, a 10.7% increase; brain and nervous system, a 30.5% increase; and non-Hodgkin's lymphoma, a 19.2% increase. The magnitude of the increases over a relatively short time, as well as the fact that rates in whites and blacks and in boys and girls alike are increasing, suggests that environmental/occupational exposures rather than generational or cohort effects over longer periods may be playing an important role in this increase.

The relationship between occupational exposures of parents and childhood cancer risks has been a topic of research interest for approximately two decades, beginning with an article by Fabia and Thuy[7] in 1974, and has been reviewed in several publications.[14,41,48,49,56] In this chapter, we will attempt to update this area of research interest, particularly highlighting the role of parental ionizing and nonionizing radiation exposures, parental chemical exposures, and the methodologic concerns that arise in such studies and how they affect the derivation of causal inferences from such studies.

METHODOLOGIC ISSUES

When one reviews the literature on the role of parental occupational exposures in risk of childhood cancer, the results may appear at first glance to be disparate and inconsistent. However, consideration of the methodologic differences of the extant studies reveals that not only are the methods used very different but that some of the methods may bias the results enough that those studies should be given less consideration in evaluating such risks. A number of methodologic issues will be considered here: selection of cases, the rationale for combining or separating cancer types, and selection of controls; sample size; timing of parental occupational exposures and latency; source of information regarding parental occupational exposures and validation of parental occupational exposures or histories; control for confounding variables and consideration of interaction; and interpretation of multiple comparisons.

Selection of Cases

Due to the rare occurrence of childhood cancer, the vast majority of studies have used the case-control design. Thus, the first step in most studies is the definition and identification of cases for study. Many of the early studies and some of the more recent studies identified cases from death certificates;[7,26,33,47,55,63] other and particularly later studies identified incident cases from hospitals serving a defined population[4,14,22,24,32,35,36,64-66] or from population-based registries.[8,15,17,21,29,34,39,42,43,46,53,59,60] As treatment and survival for childhood cancers have improved and mortality has declined,[1] the selection of cases from death records has become increasingly inappropriate, since these cases are no longer representative of the majority of childhood cancer cases, and any relationship of exposures may be more related to severity of or survival from cancer (which could be influenced by parental occupation affecting access to care) than occurrence of cancers.[48]

Furthermore, different studies include different age groups of children with cancer, which could account for some of the disparity in findings. The etiology of cancers may differ by age, with cases in younger children, for example, perhaps being more likely to be genetic[60] and cases that occur later being more likely to be due to environmental agents.

In addition, a number of studies have examined the relationship of parental occupational exposures to all cancers, rather than to specific malignancies or even to particular cell types of tumors, which may be more relevant. Often, all cancers are included in order to improve sample size and statistical power of the study. However, while relatively little is known about risk factors for specific childhood cancers, the differences in the descriptive epidemiology of specific childhood cancers, as well as knowledge about genetic-related versus spontaneous tumors, suggest that the loss of specificity achieved by studying all cancers would likely dilute any true associations[41] and thus ultimately reduce the effective statistical power of the study. One could indeed argue that from a biological perspective research should be focusing on specific histologic types of tumors to determine risk, which could differ by cell type, rather than taking the opposite approach of including all tumor types of all cancers.

Selection of Controls

The types of controls used in studies of parental occupational exposures and childhood cancer have varied greatly: from children who died from or had other illnesses, to friends or siblings, to birth certificate-matched controls. Concern about the nature of the control group arises if the selection of controls may be related to exposure, which, in the case of parental occupation, can occur. If the exposure is related to other disease conditions, or if duration of residence (which may be related to parental occupation) requirements differ for cases and controls, the potential for selection bias playing a role in the findings must be seriously considered, with relation to other conditions biasing toward the null and residence duration requirements possibly tending to bias toward a positive association. [41] This is also true if friends, siblings, or random-digit-dialed (matched on telephone prefix) controls are selected, since these groups may be more similar to cases on parental occupation, thus minimizing the chance of detecting a difference.

Sample Size

Since childhood cancer is rare, most studies have relatively few cases, particularly if only one type of malignancy is studied, and thus have relatively low statistical power for detecting differences. This problem is highlighted in the rare cohort study in which thousands of children followed over decades result in relatively few cancers of all types.[31] The problem of small sample size and low statistical power is further complicated by the fact that any one type of occupation or occupational exposure is likely to occur in only a small proportion of the subjects, thus further reducing the statistical power so that even a fairly large effect may not be statistically significant. The limitations of small sample size argue for future research on the role of parental occupation to include collaborative multicenter studies[13] with standardized protocols.

Timing of Exposures and Latency

Relatively few studies of the role of parental occupational exposures in the risk of childhood cancer have attempted to relate the timing of exposure to the risk to determine the latency period from exposure to onset of disease and to determine the period of highest risk. Many of the early studies examined parental occupation at the time of birth or diagnosis or death of the affected child,[7,17,26,29,33,47,53,55,63-65] presumably assuming that this was the relevant exposure time or that this exposure reflected exposure at the relevant time. In some recent reports, the period of exposure was not specified or was so extended that it obscured latency or period of highest risk and might have obscured or diluted associations.[21,31] However, some recent studies have attempted to determine whether preconceptional, prenatal, or postnatal exposures are associated with greatest risk.[2,4,32,34,42,59,66] Specification of the period of exposure and determination of latency are important for discerning biological mechanisms, which are currently largely only speculative, that underly any detected increased risk. Thus, such specificity is necessary to discern whether maternal or paternal preconceptional exposures alter genetic material expressed in the offspring, or if maternal prenatal exposures or paternal prenatal exposures brought home reflect transplacental carcinogenicity, or if postnatal exposures directly affect cancer risk of the offspring.

Source of Occupational Exposure Information

The sources of parental occupations and exposures have varied greatly and may account for some of the variability in findings regarding the role of parental occupational exposures in risk of childhood cancer. Sources have included birth certificates,[7,26,29,33,53,55,62-65] death certificates,[47] clinic records,[15,17] parental and surrogate interviews or questionnaires,[2-5,8,14,19,24,34,36,37,39,43,45,46, 59,60,66,67] and union records.[31]

Medical records and birth and death certificates tend to be unbiased but may result in misclassification of exposure information, which tends to direct the results toward the null, particularly if the timing of the inferred exposure is inappropriate. However, interviews and questionnaires could result in recall bias, which could bias the results away from the null.

These considerations are particularly important in interpreting the variability in study results, because virtually none of the studies have incorporated any validation of recorded or reported occupations or occupational exposures. Such an endeavor would be considerable in a case-control study, since so many different occupations in different industries in different periods of time would be recorded or reported. Most studies have made inferences about parental occupational exposures based on knowledge about occupation and/or industry in which parents worked, often using a job-exposure matrix[20] or job-exposure clusters,[23] which in turn are based on assessments by industrial hygienists of the likely presence and magnitude of exposures and combinations of exposures. Such assessments are likely to be objective and more specific than assessments of risk based only on occupation or industry, the latter being more prone to misclassification, which could result in bias toward the null. It is interesting to note, as Savitz and Chen[49] have, that even in studies in which parental occupation has been ascertained from both birth certificates and personal interviews, a determination of the reproducibility or comparability of these two sources has not been addressed.

Control for Confounding and Examination of Interaction

Since relatively little is known regarding etiologic factors for specific childhood cancers, controlling for confounding factors is somewhat of a secondary issue to those mentioned above and generally has not substantially changed results,[49] since confounding is most likely to bias the results when the confounder is a strong risk factor for the disease being studied. Nonetheless, the ability to identify and control potentially confounding factors is largely determined by the source of data for the study; clinic records and birth and death certificates provide less information about potential confounders (usually only demographic factors), and interviews and questionnaires generally provide greater access to such information. An additional consideration, however, is that some parental occupational exposures that are associated with increased risk of childhood cancer may also be correlated with each other, and each may enhance or modify the effect of another. In addition, genetic-environmental interaction could exist and would be important to consider, not only for better estimating risks but also for potentially shedding new light on potential biologic mechanisms. Few, if any, studies reported to date have attempted to investigate such interactive relationships.

Multiple Comparisons

As mentioned, virtually all of the studies of the risk of childhood cancer in relation to parental occupational exposures have been case-control in design and only one cohort study[31] has been conducted of parental occupation and childhood cancer risk. Thus, by their very nature, these case-control studies have largely involved consideration and testing of the relationship of a number of occupations, industries, and exposures to the risk of childhood cancer. Since the number of statistically significant findings is directly related to the number of significance tests performed, as well as the sample size, the possibility of some findings being statistically significant by chance alone is likely to be enhanced by this design. Therefore, when reviewing the results of a number of studies, it is important to consider the number of statistical tests performed and the sample size in each, as well as the magnitude and consistency of the measured risks across studies.

PARENTAL OCCUPATIONAL EXPOSURE TO CHEMICALS

The design and results of the studies that have reported on risks of childhood cancer associated with a number of specific parental occupational chemical exposures are summarized in Tables 1–5, and statistically significant results are noted in the footnotes. Each table reviews the studies reporting on a specific type of exposure and separates the results by type of cancer. It is hoped that this approach will be helpful in beginning to sort out some of the apparently inconsistent results and the role that differences in design may have played in differences in results. However, while each of the five tables reviews a specific exposure (manufacturing chemicals, including hydrocarbons, solvents, petroleum, paints; farming and agriculture; metals; textiles; and wood, paper and pulp), these are somewhat artificial separations that reflect specific research interests over the past two decades. For example, interest in farming and agricultural occupations has largely evolved from interest in pesticides but may well involve exposure to hydrocarbons. Machinists and miners may be exposed to hydrocarbons as well as metals. Workers in lumber and pulp mill and paper products may be exposed to hydrocarbons as well as wood products and dust. Textile workers may also have exposure to hydrocarbons. Thus, the occupations and exposures separated by and reviewed in these tables may well actually represent considerable overlap in exposures.

Hydrocarbons, Solvents, Petroleum Products, and Paints

As shown in Table 1, much of the research on parental occupational exposures and childhood cancer risks has focused on hydrocarbon-related occupations, such as machinists, drivers, service station attendants, painters, miners, printers, rubber workers, aircraft workers, and freight and transportation workers. Workers in these occupations tend to have exposures to solvents, petroleum products, and paints and dyes.

Of the nine reports that examined all cancers, which were diverse in their designs, only three had risk estimates in excess of one, two of which showed statistically significant results[17,42] for relatively nonspecific occupations, such as factory worker, manufacturing, or chemical production. More than one study was available only for leukemias and lymphomas, brain and nervous system tumors, and urinary tract tumors. Thus, this discussion will focus only on these three outcomes for discussion of these exposures.

Of the 18 studies reviewed for leukemias and lymphomas, eight reported statistically significant relationships, five of which reflected paternal occupations involving motor vehicles and transportation,[7,17,34,36,60] with times of exposure ranging from 1 year prior to birth of the child to the postnatal period and outcomes including only leukemias or only lymphomas. Of 20 studies of associations with childhood brain and nervous system tumors, three quarters reported risk estimates in excess of one, 10 of which were statistically significant results. Most of these results also relate to paternal occupations in the transportation and aircraft industries, but they also relate to painting and printing industries and to associations with hydrocarbon exposures. Most of the studies reflect the fathers'

TABLE 1. Parental Exposures to Manufacturing Chemicals (hydrocarbons, solvents, petroleum, paint) and Risk of Childh Cancer: Review of Studies

Reference	Number of Cases	Age (Years)	Incident/Dead Cases	Source of Controls	Maternal/Paternal Exposure	Time of Exposure	Type of Exposure Information	Findings	Potential Confounders Considered
All Cancers									
Fabia & Thuy[7]	386	<5	D	Birth certificates	P	At birth	Occupation on child's birth certificate	OR* = 2.1 for HCR* occupations (motor vehicle mechanic, machinist, miner, painter)	Parental age, residence, child's birthdate
Hakulinen, Salonen, & Teppo[15]	852	<15	I	Birth in same welfare district	P	At conception	Occupation in antenatal record	NSA* with HCR occupation	Child's birthdate, clinic
Kwa & Fine[33]	692	<15	D	Birth certificates	P	At birth	Occupation on child's birth certificate	NSA with HCR occupation	Child's birthdate, race and sex, and parental age
Zack, Cannon, & Loyd[67]	296	<16	I	Parents of clinic children without cancer, siblings of case parents, and neighbors	M & P	Year before birth, year after birth, year before diagnosis, entire interval before diagnosis	Industry and occupation from parental interviews	NSA with father motor vehicle mechanic, service station attendant, machinist, miner, lumberman, painter, dyer, cleaner; NSA with maternal HCR occupations	Parental age and education, child's age, gender and race
Hemminki, Saloniemi, & Salonen[17]	1700	<15	I	Birth in same welfare district	M & P	During pregnancy	Occupation in antenatal record	OR† = 2.29 for maternal factory worker; OR = 2.75† for paternal occupation as painter	Child's birthdate, parental age, maternal parity, and child's birthweight
Sanders, White, & Draper[47]	20	<15	D	Childhood deaths	P	At child's death	Occupation on child's death certificate	NSA with HCR occupations	Social class

Reference	N	Age	Design	Control source	Parent	Timing	Exposure assessment	Results	Adjustments
Olsen, de Nully Brown, Schulgen, & Jensen[42]	1721	<15	I	Population register	M & P	At conception	Job title, company, and industry in pension fund records	OR = 1.15† for paternal manufacturing; OR = 3.1† for paternal production of chemicals; OR = 3.3† for paternal work in technical and chemical laboratories	Child's sex and date of birth, parental age
Feingold, Savitz, & John[8]	252	<15	I	Random-digit dialing	M & P	Year prior to birth	Job title and industry from parental interview used in job-exposure matrix[20]	NSA with maternal or paternal HCR occupations; OR = 1.9 for maternal benzene exposure; OR = 2.1 for maternal petroleum/coke pitch/tar exposure; OR = 3.3 for maternal soot exposure; OR = 2.5 for paternal creosote exposure; OR = 2.0 for paternal polysiloxane exposure;	Child's age and sex, telephone exchange, paternal education, maternal smoking
Kristensen & Andersen[31]	7++ 25	<15 >14	I	Oslo incidence rates	P	Preconception	Union records for printers	SIR* = 0.50 for cases <14 yrs; SIR = 1.04 for cases <14 yrs for all printers; SIR = 0.35 for solvent exposure for cases <14 yrs	Child's gender and age and calendar year of diagnosis

Leukemias and Lymphomas

Reference	N	Age	Design	Control source	Parent	Timing	Exposure assessment	Results	Adjustments
Fabia & Thuy[7]	218	<5	D	Birth certificates	P	At birth	Occupation on child's birth certificate	OR = 1.9† for motor vehicle mechanics/service station attendants; OR = 2.5† for machinist/miner/lumberman	Parental age, residence, child's birthdate

(Continued on next page)

TABLE 1.   Parental Exposures to Manufacturing Chemicals (hydrocarbons, solvents, petroleum, paint) and Risk of Childhood Cancer: Review of Studies (*Continued*)

Reference	Number of Cases	Age (Years)	Incident/ Dead Cases	Source of Controls	Maternal/ Paternal Exposure	Time of Exposure	Type of Exposure Information	Findings	Potential Confounders Considered
Hakulinen, Salonen, & Teppo[15]	339	<15	I	Birth in same welfare district	P	At conception	Occupation in antenatal record	OR = 0.91 for motor vehicle mechanic, service station attendant, miner, machinist, lumberman, painter, dyer, cleaner, or driver	Child's birthdate, clinic
Kwa & Fine[33]	430	<15	D	Birth certificates	P	At birth	Occupation on child's birth certificate	NSA with HCR occupations	Child's birthdate, sex and race, parental age
Zack, Cannon, & Loyd, et al.[67]	158	<16	I	Parents of clinic children without cancer, siblings of case parents, and neighbors	P	Year before birth, year after birth, year before diagnosis, entire interval before diagnosis	Occupation and industry from parental interviews	NSA with paternal HCR occupations	Parental age and education, child's age, gender and race
Hemminki, Saloniemi, & Salonen[17]	319	<15	I[a]	Birth in same welfare district	M & P	During pregnancy	Occupation in antenatal record	OR = 1.33 for maternal factory worker; OR = 1.90[†] for paternal motor vehicle drivers	Child's birthdate, parental age, maternal parity and child's birthweight
Sanders, White, & Draper[47]	2771	<15	D[a]	Childhood deaths	P	At child's death	Occupation on child's death certificate	PMR* = 92.5 for HCR occupation	Social class

Study	N	Age	Grade	Control source	M/P	Exposure timing	Exposure assessment	Results	Variables controlled
Gold, Diener, & Szklo[14]	43	<20	I[a]	Other childhood cancers and birth certificates	P	Before birth, between birth and diagnosis	Occupation from maternal interviews	OR = 0.83–3.0 for HCR occupations before birth; OR = 1.29–1.60 for HCR occupations between birth and diagnosis	Child's sex, race, and age
Shaw, Lavey, Jackson, et al.[53]	255	<16	I[a]	Birth certificate	P	At birth	Occupation on child's birth certificate	NSA with paternal benzene exposure	Child's sex and season and year of birth, county of birth
Vianna, Kovasznay, Polan, et al.[60]	60	<1	I[a]	Birth certificate	P	At least one year prior to birth	Occupation from maternal interview	OR = 2.4†–2.5† for high motor exhaust exposure; OR = 1.3–3.8† for low motor exhaust exposure; significant association for high exhaust exposure in female but not male cases	Child's year of birth, sex, race, county of residence, maternal age, birth order
Van Steensel-Moll, Valkenburg, & Van Zanen[59]	519	<15	I[b]	Same census region as case	M & P	During pregnancy and one year before diagnosis	Occupation from parental interviews	NSA with paternal HCR occupations; OR = 2.5 for maternal HCR occupations during pregnancy; OR = 2.4† for maternal chemical exposure during pregnancy; OR = 1.8 for maternal pigment/dye exposure during pregnancy; OR = 2.0 for paternal plastic or rubber exposure; OR = 1.6 for paternal pigment/dye exposure during pregnancy	Child's date of birth and sex, place of residence at diagnosis, birth order, father's education

(Continued on next page)

TABLE 1. Parental Exposures to Manufacturing Chemicals (hydrocarbons, solvents, petroleum, paint) and Risk of Childhood Cancer: Review of Studies (Continued)

Reference	Number of Cases	Age (Years)	Incident/ Dead Cases	Source of Controls	Maternal/ Paternal Exposure	Time of Exposure	Type of Exposure Information	Findings	Potential Confounders Considered
Lowengart, Peters, Cicioni, et al.[34]	123	< 11	I[a]	Friends of case or random-digit-dialing	M & P	From one year prior to conception to one year prior to diagnosis	Occupations and exposures from maternal interviews	OR = 2.0[†] for all paternal manufacturing; OR = 2.5[†] for paternal transportation equipment manufacturing; OR = 3.0[†] for paternal machinery manufacturing; OR = 2.2[†] for paternal spray paint exposure during pregnancy and 2.0 after delivery; OR = 3.5[†] for paternal exposure to chlorinated solvents, 4.5[†] for exposure to dyes/ pigments, 1.7[†] for exposure to cutting oils, and 3.0[†] for exposure to methylethyl ketone after delivery; NSA with maternal exposure to these agents	Child's age, sex, race and Hispanic origin, and socio-economic status
Buckley, Robison, Swotinsky, et al.[2]	178	< 18	I[c]	Random-digit-dialing	M & P	From one year prior to conception to one year prior to diagnosis	Occupations and exposures from parental interviews	OR = 2.0[†]–2.6[†] for paternal exposure to solvents, 1.8–3.3[†] for exposure to plastics, 1.4–2.4[†] for exposure to petroleum products; OR = 1.5–2.2[†] for maternal exposure to paint/pigments, strongest associations for exposure before and during pregnancy	Child's date of birth and race

Reference	No.	Age	Design	Controls	M/P	Exposure period	Exposure assessment	Results	Adjustment/matching
Magnani, Pastore, Luzzatto, & Terracini[36]	183	All	I	Hospitalized children, excluding cancer, Down's syndrome, β-thalassemia, infections, mononucleosis, lymphadenitis or unexplained splenic enlargement	M & P	Up to child's birth and between birth and diagnosis	Occupations from interviews with closest relative	OR = 5.0† for lymphoma associated with paternal lorry driver; OR = 7.6–10.1† for acute nonlymphocytic leukemia associated with paternal worker in tire production	Socioeconomic status
Infante-Rivard, Mur, Armstrong, et al.[24]	128	<15	I[b]	Census	M	During pregnancy	Occupation and exposures from maternal interviews	OR = 0.62 for solvent exposure; OR = 0.50 for exposure to oil, grease, hydrocarbons	Child's year of birth, sex and municipality at diagnosis
Olsen, de Nully Brown, Schulgen, & Jensen[42]	603	<15	I	Population register	M & P	At conception	Job title, company and industry in pension records	OR = 5.8† for association of leukemia with paternal employment in rubber; 7.0† for office machine manufacture; 2.8† for machine repair workshops; OR = 14.5† for maternal employment in porcelain, 14.5† for communication material manufacture, and 3.9† for wholesale trade of raw materials	Child's sex and date of birth, parental age
Feingold, Savitz, & John[8]	59	<15	I[b]	Random-digit-dialing	P	Year prior to birth	Job title and industry from parental interview used in job exposure matrix[20]	OR = 1.3 for any paternal hydrocarbon exposure, 2.1 for aniline and anthracene, dose-response for increasing levels of exposure to petroleum/coke pitch/tar (1.2, 2.0, 2.9)	Child's age and sex, telephone exchange, paternal education, maternal smoking

(Continued on next page)

TABLE 1. Parental Exposures to Manufacturing Chemicals (hydrocarbons, solvents, petroleum, paint) and Risk of Childhood Cancer: Review of Studies (Continued)

Reference	Number of Cases	Age (Years)	Incident/ Dead Cases	Source of Controls	Maternal/ Paternal Exposure	Time of Exposure	Type of Exposure Information	Findings	Potential Confounders Considered
Kristensen & Andersen[31]	2	<15	I[a]	Oslo incidence rates	P	Preconception	Union records for printers	SIR = 0.44	Child's gender and age and calendar year of diagnosis
Roman, Watson, Beral, et al.[46]	51	<5	I	Hospital delivery registers and live birth registers	P	At birth and from 3 years before birth to diagnosis	Occupation on child's birth certificate and from parental interviews	OR = 0.6–1.3 for drivers and related occupations	Child's sex, date of birth, and area of residence at birth and diagnosis
Brain and Nervous System									
Fabia & Thuy[7]	101	<5	D	Birth certificates	P	At birth	Occupation on child's birth certificate	OR = 2.8[†] for paternal motor vehicle mechanic, service station attendant	Parental age, residence, child's birthdate
Hakulinen, Salonen, & Teppo[15]	219	<15	I	Birth in same welfare district	P	At conception	Occupation in antenatal record	OR = 0.96 for paternal motor vehicle mechanic, service station attendant, machinist, miner, lumberman, painter, dyer, cleaner, driver	Child's birthdate, clinic
Kwa & Fine[33]	132	<15	D	Birth certificates	P	At birth	Occupation on child's birth certificate	OR = 0.69 for mechanic, gas station attendant, machinist, painter, printer, driver	Child's birthdate, race, and sex, parental age
Zack, Cannon, Loyd, et al.[67]	52	<16	I	Parents of clinic children without cancer, siblings of case parents, and neighbors	P	Year before birth, year after birth, year before diagnosis, entire interval before diagnosis	Industry and occupation from parental interviews	NSA with father motor vehicle mechanic, service station attendant, machinist, miner, lumberman, painter, dyer, cleaner	Parental age and education, child's age, gender and race

Reference	N	Age	Design	Control source	Parent	Exposure period	Exposure assessment	Results	Factors controlled
Hemminki, Saloniemi, & Salonen[17]	82	<15	I[d]	Birth in same welfare district	M & P	During pregnancy	Occupation in antenatal record	OR = 8.0 for maternal factory worker; OR = 0.92–5.00[†] for paternal motor vehicle drivers or painters; OR = 4.39[†] for paternal machine repairmen	Child's birthplace, parental age, maternal parity, child's birthweight
Peters, Preston-Martin, & Yu[45]	92	<10	I[d]	Friend or neighbor	M & P	From one year before conception through lactation, or at time of diagnosis for father	Job, industry and exposures from maternal interviews	OR= 3.0[†] mother inhaled chemicals or fumes; OR = 2.8[†] for father exposed to chemical solvents; OR = 7.0[†] for father exposed to paints; OR = ∞** for father working in aircraft industry	Child's sex, race and year of birth, social class, other parent's exposures, food consumption patterns, drug use, alcohol use, smoking
Sanders, White, & Draper[47]	1,921	<15	D[d]	Childhood deaths	P	At child's death	Occupation on child's death certificate	PMR = 91–95 for HCR occupations	Social class
Gold, Diener, & Szklo[14]	70	<20	I[d]	Other childhood cancers, birth certificates	P	Before birth, between birth and diagnosis	Occupation from maternal interview	OR = 0.54–2.3 for HCR occupation before birth; OR = 0.77–4.0[†] for HCR occupation between birth and diagnosis	Child's sex, race and age
Olshan, Breslow, Daling, et al.[43]	51	<16	I[d]	Random-digit-dialing	P	Year prior to birth, from year prior to birth to diagnosis	Occupation and industry from parental interviews	OR = 0.66 for employment in aerospace in year prior to birth; OR = 0.53 for aerospace employment from year prior to birth to diagnosis; OR = 0–2.51 for aerospace employment any time, stratified by age	Child's age, sex and race, parental age, smoking, drinking, and maternal exposure to chemicals

(Continued on next page)

TABLE 1. Parental Exposures to Manufacturing Chemicals (hydrocarbons, solvents, petroleum, paint) and Risk of Childhood Cancer: Review of Studies (*Continued*)

Reference	Number of Cases	Age (Years)	Incident/ Dead Cases	Source of Controls	Maternal/ Paternal Exposure	Time of Exposure	Type of Exposure Information	Findings	Potential Confounders Considered
Spitz & Johnson[55]	157	<15	D[e]	Birth certificate	P	At birth	Occupation and industry on birth certificate used in job-exposure clusters[23]	NSA with HCR occupations; OR = 3.17[†] for aromatic and aliphatic hydrocarbon exposure cluster	Child's birth year
Johnson, Annegers, & Frankowski[26]	499	<15	D	Birth certificate	P	At birth	Occupation and industry on birth certificate	OR = 0.7–1.5 for HCR occupations; OR = 4.5[†] for printing; OR = 21.9[†] for graphic artists; OR = 5.1[†] for newspaper and printing industry; OR = 0.8–3.0[†] for chemical and petroleum industry	Child's birthdate, race, and sex
Nasca, Baptiste, MacCubbin, et al.[39]	338	<15	I	Birth certificates	P	At birth, at diagnosis	Occupation and industry from maternal interviews	OR = 1.11–1.41 for HCR occupation at birth or diagnosis; OR = 3.14[†] for petroleum industry employment at birth; OR = 0.57–1.49 for aircraft or chemical industry employment at birth; OR = 0.29–1.72 for petroleum, chemical, or aircraft industry employment at diagnosis	Child's age, sex, and race

Wilkins & Koutras[63]	491	<20	D[d]	Birth certificate	P	At birth	Industry and occupation on birth certificate used in job-exposure matrix[20]	OR = 1.6†–1.9 for employment in chemical, drugs, paint, and transportation industries; OR = 0.9–5.9 for printers, mechanics and machine repairers, miners, painters, plasterers, and related occupations	Child's age, race, sex, birth order, and birthweight, parental age, and proportion of farmland in county of residence
Howe, Burch, Chiarelli, et al[22]	74	<20	I[d]	Population lists	M & P	"Usual occupation"	Occupation from maternal interviews	OR = 0.08–3.7 for paternal painters, drivers, printers, machinists, mechanics, or factory worker; OR = 5.03† for maternal factory worker	Child's sex and date of birth and area of residence
Wilkins & Sinks[66]	110	<20	I[d]	Random-digit-dialing	M & P	Preconception, prenatal, postnatal periods	Occupation and industry from parental interviews used in job-exposure matrix[20] and job exposure clusters[23]	OR = 1.7–2.3 for paternal motor freight and transportation occupation during the 3 periods; OR = 0.7–1.8 for paternal work in machinery, transportation, rubber, plastics, synthetics, and fuel industries; OR = 2.6 for maternal occupation in processing OR = 0.8–1.6 for maternal work in machinery industry; OR = 1.5–7.0† for paternal exposure to hydrocarbons, highest ORs in prenatal and preconception periods; OR = 1.7–2.2 for maternal hydrocarbon exposures	Child's year of birth, race, and sex

(Continued on next page)

TABLE 1. Parental Exposures to Manufacturing Chemicals (hydrocarbons, solvents, petroleum, paint) and Risk of Childhood Cancer: Review of Studies (*Continued*)

Reference	Number of Cases	Age (Years)	Incident/ Dead Cases	Source of Controls	Maternal/ Paternal Exposure	Time of Exposure	Type of Exposure Information	Findings	Potential Confounders Considered
Bunin, Petrakova, Meadows, et al.[5]	104	All	I[e]	Random-digit-dialing	M & P	Preconception and prenatal	Occupation and company from parental interviews used in job exposure matrix[20] and job-exposure clusters[23]	OR = 0.8–2.0 for paternal exposure clusters in electrical equipment, rubber processing, and printing; OR = 1.3–2.0 for paternal chemistry occupation and tire manufacturing	Child's race, birthdate, and telephone exchange
Olsen, de Nully Brown, Schulgen, & Jensen[42]	416	< 15	I	Population register	M & P	At conception	Job title, company and industry in pension fund records	OR = 7.0[†] for paternal employment in chemical raw materials industry; OR = 5.9[†] for paternal employment in auto repair	Child's sex and date of birth, parental age
Feingold, Savitz, & John[8]	67	< 15	I[d]	Random-digit-dialing	P	Year prior to birth	Job title and industry from parental interview used in job exposure matrix[20]	OR = 0.7–3.7 for paternal hydrocarbon exposures	Child's age and sex, telephone exchange, paternal education, maternal smoking
Kristensen & Andersen[31]	2, 4	≤ 14, > 14	I	Oslo incidence rates	P	Preconception	Union records for printers	SIR = 0.49 for age ≤ 14 and 1.33 for age > 14 yrs for paternal printer	Child's gender and age and year of diagnosis

Study	N	Age	Design	Source	M & P	Time period	Exposure assessment	Results	Adjustment/matching
Kuitjen, Bunin, Nass, & Meadows[32]	163	<15	I^d	Random-digit-dialing	M & P	Preconception, prenatal, and postnatal periods	Job title and industry from parental interviews	OR = 1.0–1.7 for paternal work in chemical industry; OR = 1.2–1.5 for paternal work in newspaper and printing industry; OR = 0–0.2 for paternal work in aerospace; OR = 0.6–1.3 for paternal chemical and petroleum occupation; OR = 2.5–4.0 for paternal printer	Child's age, race and telephone area code
Urinary Tract Cancers									
Kantor, Curnen, Meigs, et al.[29]	149	<19	I^f	Birth certificates	P	At birth	Occupation on child's birth certificate	OR = 2.4† for HCR occupations; OR = 1.7 for machinists; OR = 6.0 for motor vehicle mechanics	Child's sex, race, and year of birth
Kwa & Fine[33]	34	<15	D	Birth certificates	P	At birth	Occupation on child's birth certificate	OR = 2.5† for paternal mechanics, gas station attendant, machinist	Child's birthdate, race, and sex, parental age
Zack, Cannon, Loyd, et al.[67]	27	<16	I^f	Parents of clinic children, siblings of case parents, and neighbors	M & P	Years before birth, years after birth, year before diagnosis, entire interval before diagnosis	Occupation and industry from parental interviews	OR = 1.46–∞ for paternal machinist, miner, lumberman	Parental age and education, child's age, gender, and race
Sanders, White, & Draper[47]	398	<15	D^f	Childhood deaths	P	At child's death	Occupation on child's death certificate	PMR = 114–119 for HCR occupations	Social class

(Continued on next page)

TABLE 1. Parental Exposures to Manufacturing Chemicals (hydrocarbons, solvents, petroleum, paint) and Risk of Childhood Cancer: Review of Studies (*Continued*)

Reference	Number of Cases	Age (Years)	Incident/ Dead Cases	Source of Controls	Maternal/ Paternal Exposure	Time of Exposure	Type of Exposure Information	Findings	Potential Confounders Considered
Wilkins & Sinks[64]	62	All	I[f]	Birth certificates	P	At birth	Occupation and industry on birth certificate used for job exposure matrix[20]	OR = 0.80–2.19 for machinery industry; OR = 1.51 for transportation industry; OR = 0.48 for motor and freight and transportation occupations; OR = 4.0 for brake fluids, alicyclic hydrocarbons, rubber, oils, chlorinated benzene	Child's age, sex, race, and maternal county of residence
Wilkins & Sinks[65]	62	All	I[f]	Birth certificates	P	At birth	Occupation on child's birth certificate	OR = 1.37–1.40 for HCR occupations; OR = 6.0 for painters	Child's race, sex, and year of birth and maternal county of residence
Bunin, Nass, Kramer, & Meadows[4]	88 (whites only)	<15	I[f]	Random-digit-dialing	M & P	Preconception, prenatal, birth to 6 mos. prior to diagnosis	Job and industry from parental interviews used in job exposure matrix[20] and job exposure clusters[23]	OR = 4.2†–5.0† for paternal exposure to aromatic or aliphatic hydrocarbons in preconception or prenatal periods (most excess risk for "genetic" cases); NSA with maternal exposures	Child's race, date of birth and telephone area code and prefix, proxy interview
Olsen, de Nully Brown, Schulgen, & Jensen[42]	132	<15	I[f]	Population register	M & P	At conception	Job title, company, and industry in pension fund records	OR = 1.5† for paternal manufacturing work	Child's sex and date of birth, parental age

Soft Tissue Sarcoma (STS) and Rhabdomyosarcoma (RMS)

Study	No.	Age		Controls	M & P	Exposure Window	Exposure Assessment	Results	Matching/Adjustment
Magnani, Pastore, Luzzatto, et al.[35]	52 STS and 36 RMS	All	I	Hospitalized children without cancer, Down's syndrome, β-thalassemia, infectious mononucleosis, lymphadenitis, or unspecified splenic enlargement	M & P	Before birth and birth to diagnosis	Occupation from interviews with close relatives	OR = 5.4[†] for motor machine tool operator before birth; OR = 4.8[†] for father in appliance production before birth	Clinical center

Retinoblastoma

Study	No.	Age		Controls	M & P	Exposure Window	Exposure Assessment	Results	Matching/Adjustment
Bunin, Petrakova, Meadows, et al.[5]	201	All	I	Random-digit-dialing	M & P	Preconception, postconception	Occupation from parental interviews used in job-exposure matrix[20] and job exposure clusters[23]	NSA for parental HCR occupations and sporadic cases	Child's date of birth, race, and telephone area code and first five digits of phone number

Hepatoblastoma

Study	No.	Age		Controls	M & P	Exposure Window	Exposure Assessment	Results	Matching/Adjustment
Buckley, Sather, Ruccione, et al.[3]	75	All	I	Random-digit-dialing	M & P	Ever	Occupations and exposures from parental interviews	OR = 0.7–1.5 for parental exposure to solvents, cleaning agents, plastics; OR = 3.7[†] for maternal exposure to paints, pigment or oil or coal products; OR = 1.5–1.9 for paternal exposure to paints, pigments or oil or coal products	Child's age, other chemical exposures

Benign and Malignant Germ Cell Tumors

Study	No.	Age		Controls	M & P	Exposure Window	Exposure Assessment	Results	Matching/Adjustment
Johnston, Mann, Williams, et al.[28]	41	<15	I	General practitioner and hospital lists of patients with non-neoplastic disease	M & P	Year prior to pregnancy	Exposures from parental interviews	OR = 1.74–4.73 for maternal exposure to dusts and chemicals; OR = 2.92–6.55 for paternal exposure to dusts and chemicals	Child's age and gender

* Abbreviations: OR = odds ratio; NSA = no significant association; PMR = proportionate mortality ratio; SIR = standardized incidence ratio; HCR = hydrocarbon-related (includes factory worker, machinist, driver, motor vehicle mechanic, service station attendant, miner, lumberman, painter, dry cleaner).

[†] $p < 0.05$　　　†† cohort study of 10,829 children

** $p < 0.001$

[a] leukemias only; [b] acute lymphocytic leukemia only; [c] acute nonlymphocytic leukemia only; [d] brain tumors only; [e] neuroblastoma only; [f] Wilms' tumor only.

occupations at the time of birth of the child, although some report on more extensive periods. Of the eight studies reviewed relating to urinary tract cancers, all found risk estimates in excess of one, and four studies showed statistically significant results, most of which were for paternal hydrocarbon-related occupations any time from prior to conception to six months prior to diagnosis of the child's cancer. Thus the evidence for increased risk of brain and nervous system tumors and urinary tract cancers associated with paternal occupational hydrocarbon exposure represents perhaps some of the most consistent results.

Farming and Agricultural Occupations and Exposures

Most of the findings of the four studies that were reviewed for all cancers combined showed no significant association with farming or agricultural occupations or exposures (Table 2). Only in the study by Hemminki et al.[17] was there a nonstatistically significant association of maternal occupation in agriculture, gardening, or forestry during pregnancy (OR = 1.73 for 1959–75 and OR = 2.16 for 1969–75) and for fathers only during the early part of the study period (OR = 1.42, p = 0.05 for 1959–68). Of the seven studies that investigated associations with leukemias and lymphomas, four reported risk estimates in excess of one, three of which showed statistically significant excesses either with maternal or paternal exposure to pesticides particularly during and after pregnancy[2,34] or with paternal work in wholesale agricultural machinery.[42] Of the seven studies reviewed for associations with brain and nervous system tumors, five showed positive associations, only two of which showed statistically significant excesses for paternal work in the agriculture, forestry, or fishing industry at the time of birth of the index child[63] or for paternal work in dairies or maternal work in slaughterhouses or meat packing at the time of conception of the index child.[42] For urinary tract cancers, only two studies were reviewed, both by the same authors on the same study group, and both showed no association with Wilms' tumor. Only one study reported a large, statistically significant positive association of Ewing's bone sarcoma with paternal occupation in agriculture or paternal exposure to pesticides, herbicides, or fertilizers,[21] although one other study that did separate out bone sarcomas in its analyses did not report any significant associations with agricultural occupations or exposures.[42] Thus, it would appear that there is no overwhelming or strongly consistent evidence for an association of any tumor site with parental agricultural occupations or exposures.

Metals

Only 13 studies have reported on associations of parental occupational metal exposure with risk either of all types or any specific type of childhood cancer (Table 3). Ten reported positive associations, and seven showed statistically significant associations. Perhaps the most consistent findings are for associations with brain and nervous system tumors, for which three of the five studies reviewed found statistically significant associations with welding or the metal industry either at the time of birth of the index child or preconceptionally.[55,63,66] Also worthy of note were two of four studies reporting positive associations of paternal work at conception or prenatally in metal manufacturing with Wilms' tumor,[4,42] as well as one study showing a statistically significant association of paternal metal work and retinoblastoma[5] and one study showing statistically significant associations of maternal and paternal occupations in metal with hepatoblastoma.[3]

Textiles

While relatively few studies have reported on associations of work in textiles with risk of childhood cancer (Table 4), three of four studies on such an association with leukemias and lymphomas have reported statistically significant associations for maternal and paternal exposures particularly during pregnancy.[24,36,59] Studies of an association with brain and nervous system cancers have largely been inconsistent. However, one additional study has reported significant associations for soft tissue sarcomas with maternal and paternal work in textiles before the birth of the index child.[35]

Wood, Paper and Pulp

While no association has been reported between wood, paper, and pulp-related occupations and all cancers combined (Table 5), two of four studies that have examined the relationship to leukemias and lymphomas have found statistically significant associations with maternal or paternal work in construction or in wood-related occupations.[36,42] Further, of seven studies investigating such an association with childhood brain and nervous system tumors, six have found positive associations, two of which found statistically significant associations with paternal work in construction at the time of birth of the index child[13] or in carpentry at conception of the child.[42] The latter study also reported a significant association of paternal work in the wood and furniture industry at conception with risk of Wilms' tumor, and one other study[36] reported a significant association of paternal work in the building industry postnatally with risk of soft tissue sarcoma.

PARENTAL PRECONCEPTION OCCUPATIONAL EXPOSURE TO PHYSICAL AGENTS

Studies of childhood cancers have examined the evidence of associations of selected types of cancer, or all cancers, with parental preconception exposure to physical agents. The majority of studies have evaluated associations with paternal occupational exposures. Particular attention has focused on both ionizing and nonionizing radiation in the form of extremely low electromagnetic fields (EMF). Several aspects of these studies are worth emphasizing.

The first point is that for physical agents, unlike chemicals or drugs, male-mediated effects must be direct through modification of the sperm. For chemicals, male effects through chemical contamination of clothing brought into the house or chemicals in semen are possible. This is not the case with physical agents.

A related point is that a direct male-mediated effect must be either via a transmissible genetic effect or a sperm-determined epigenetic effect. A transmissible genetic effect requires a mutational event to occur—for instance, the agent must be mutagen, either altering the structure of a chromosome or of an individual gene or genes. While epigenetic mechanisms, such as imprinting, may be relevant, this is a relatively new area of research.[44]

Finally, studies of workers occupationally exposed to ionizing radiation often have the advantage of having quantified exposure data available from dosimetric records. This allows the determination of individual, and often time-specific, doses. Depending on the source of records, these data are often available for various types of whole body penetrating radiation and for internal emitters (radionuclides) as well.

TABLE 2. Parental Exposures Related to Farming and Agriculture and Risk of Childhood Cancer: Review of Studies

Reference	Number of Cases	Age (Years)	Incident/ Dead Cases	Source of Controls	Maternal/ Paternal Exposure	Time of Exposure	Type of Exposure Information	Findings	Potential Confounders Considered
All Cancers									
Zack, Cannon, Loyd, et al.[67]	296	<16	I	Parents of clinic children without cancer, siblings of case parents, and neighbors	M & P	Year before birth, year after birth, year before diagnosis, entire interval before diagnosis	Industry and occupation from parental interviews	NSA* with fathers as farmers	Parental age and education, child's age, gender, and race
Hemminki, Saloniemi, & Salonen[17]	1,700	<15	I	Birth in same welfare district	M & P	During pregnancy	Occupation in antenatal record	OR* = 0.8–2.16 for mother in agriculture, gardening, or forestry; OR = 1.05–1.42† for father in agriculture, gardening, or forestry; OR = 1.22 for paternal farmers	Child's birthdate, parental age, maternal parity, child's birthweight
Sanders, White, & Draper[47]	6,920	<15	D	Childhood deaths	P	At child's death	Occupation on child's death certificate	PMR* = 109–121 for farmers	Social class
Olsen, de Nully Brown, Schulgen, & Jensen[42]	1,721	<15	I	Population register	M & P	At conception	Job title, company, and industry in pension fund records	OR = 0.79–0.89 for parents in farming, forestry, or fishery	Child's sex and date of birth, parental age
Leukemias and Lymphomas									
Hemminki, Saloniemi, & Salonen[17]	319	<15	I[a]	Birth in same welfare district	M & P	During pregnancy	Occupation in antenatal record	OR = 1.26 for paternal farmers	Child's birthdate, parental age, maternal parity, child's birthweight

Reference	No.		Controls	M & P	Exposure period	Exposure assessment	Results	Matching variables
Van-Steensel-Moll, Valkenburg, Van Zanen[59]	519	I[b]	Same census region as case	M & P	During pregnancy, one year before diagnosis	Occupation from parental interviews	OR = 0.4–0.9 for mother or father in agriculture, forestry, and horti-culture; OR = 0.7–1.0 for parental exposure to pesticides, herbicides, and insecticides	Child's date of birth and sex, place of residence at diagnosis, birth order, father's education
Lowengart, Peters, Cicioni, et al.[34]	123	I[a]	Friends of case or random-digit-dialing	M & P	One year pre-conception to one year pre-diagnosis	Occupations and exposures from maternal interviews	OR = 1.0 for father in agriculture; OR = 5.0–9.0[†] for parent exposed to garden pesticides or herbicides ≥ once a month during pregnancy	Child's age, sex, race, and Hispanic origin and socioeconomic status
Buckley, Robison, Swotinsky, et al.[2]	178	I[c]	Random-digit-dialing	M & P	One year preconception to one year prediagnosis	Occupations and exposures from parental interviews	OR = 1.02–2.7[†] for paternal exposure to pesticides (trend $p = 0.06$); OR = 1.0–∞[†] for maternal exposure to pesticides (trend $p = 0.008$); particularly associated during and after pregnancy, all ages and m4/m5 morphology	Child's date of birth and race
Infante-Rivard, Mur, Armstrong, et al.[24]	128	I[b]	Census	M	During pregnancy	Occupation and exposures from maternal interviews	OR = 1.80 for work in agriculture; OR = 1.40 for exposure to insecticides	Child's year of birth, sex and municipality at diagnosis
Olsen, de Nully Brown, Schulgen, & Jensen[42]	603	I	Population register	M & P	At conception	Job title, company and industry in pension records	OR = 4.6[†] for father's work in wholesale agriculture machinery	Child's sex and date of birth, parental age

(Continued on next page)

TABLE 2. Parental Exposures Related to Farming and Agriculture and Risk of Childhood Cancer: Review of Studies *(Continued)*

Reference	Number of Cases	Age (Years)	Incident/ Dead Cases	Source of Controls	Maternal/ Paternal Exposure	Time of Exposure	Type of Exposure Information	Findings	Potential Confounders Considered
Roman, Watson, Beral, et al.[46]	51	<5	I	Hospital delivery registers and live birth registers	P	At birth, and from 3 years before birth to diagnosis	Occupation on child's birth certificate and from parental interviews	OR = 0.8–1.1 for agriculture	Child's sex, date of birth and area of residence at birth and diagnosis
Brain and Nervous System									
Hemminki, Saloniemi, & Salonen[17]	282	<15	I[d]	Birth in same welfare district	M & P	During pregnancy	Occupation in antenatal record	OR = 1.15 for paternal farmer	Child's birthdate, parental age, maternal parity, child's birthweight
Spitz & Johnson[55]	157	<15	D[e]	Birth certificates	P	At birth	Occupation and industry on birth certificate used in job-exposure clusters[23]	OR = 0.55 for agriculture occupation	Child's birth year
Wilkins & Koutras[63]	491	<20	D[d]	Birth certificates	P	At birth	Industry and occupation on birth certificate for job-exposure matrix[20]	OR = 2.4[†] for agriculture, forestry or fishing industry; OR = 1.8 for occupation in agriculture, fishery and forestry	Child's age, race, sex, birth order and birthweight, parental age and proportion of farmland in county of residence
Bunin, Ward, Kramer, et al.[6]	104	All	I[e]	Random-digit-dialing	M & P	Preconception and prenatal	Occupation and company from parental interviews used in job-exposure matrix[20] and job-exposure clusters[23]	OR = 0.7–3.5 for paternal farmers and agricultural workers	Child's race, birthdate, and telephone exchange

Reference	N	Age		Source	Parent	Time period	Exposure assessment	Results	Adjustment variables
Wilkins & Sinks[66]	110	<20	I[d]	Random-digit-dialing	M & P	Preconception, prenatal and postnatal periods	Occupation and industry from parental interview used in job-exposure matrix[20] and job-exposure clusters	OR = 0.9–2.7 for paternal occupation in agriculture; OR = 1.0–2.8 for paternal industry agriculture, forestry and fishing	Child's year of birth, race, and sex
Olsen, de Nully Brown, Schulgen, & Jensen[42]	416	<15	I	Population register	M & P	At conception	Job title, company and industry in pension records	OR = 3.8[†] for paternal work in dairies; OR = 7.3[†] for maternal work in slaughter house or meat packing	Child's sex and state of birth, parental age
Kuijten, Bunin, Nass, & Meadows[32]	163	<15	I[d]	Random-digit-dialing	M & P	Preconception, prenatal, and postnatal periods	Job title and industry from parental interviews	OR = 1.0–1.8 for paternal agricultural occupation	Child's age, race, and telephone area code
Urinary Tract Cancers									
Wilkins & Sinks[64]	62	All	I[f]	Birth certificates	P	At birth	Occupation and industry on birth certificate used for job-exposure matrix[20]	OR = 0.46–0.64 for agriculture industry and occupation; OR = 0.3 for exposure to insecticides	Child's age, sex and race and maternal county of residence
Wilkins & Sinks[65]	62	All	I[f]	Birth certificates	P	At birth	Occupation on child's birth certificate	OR = 0.47–0.58 for farmer	Child's race, sex, and year of birth, and maternal county of residence

(Continued on next page)

TABLE 2. Parental Exposures Related to Farming and Agriculture and Risk of Childhood Cancer: Review of Studies *(Continued)*

Reference	Number of Cases	Age (Years)	Incident/ Dead Cases	Source of Controls	Maternal/ Paternal Exposure	Time of Exposure	Type of Exposure Information	Findings	Potential Confounders Considered
Ewing's Bone Sarcoma									
Holly, Aston, Ahn, & Kristiansen[21]	43	All	I	Random-digit-dialing	M & P	Six months prior to conception to diagnosis	Occupation and exposures from maternal interview	OR = 8.8[†] for paternal agriculture occupation; OR = 6.1[†] for paternal exposure to herbicides, pesticides, or fertilizers	Child's sex and age and telephone area code and prefix, income, poison, overdose of medication
Retinoblastoma									
Bunin, Petrakova, Meadows, et al.[5]	201	All	I	Random-digit-dialing	M & P	Preconception, postconception	Occupation from parental interviews used in job-exposure matrix[20] and job-exposure clusters[23]	OR = 1.0 for maternal grandfathers of sporadic heritable cases being farmers, farm workers; OR = 10.0[†] for nonheritable cases, maternal grandfather works as farmers, farm workers; NSA of fathers with herbicide exposure	Child's date of birth, race, and telephone area code and first five digits of phone number

* Abbreviations: OR = odds ratio; NSA = no significant association; PMR = proportionate mortality ratio.
† $p < 0.05$ †† cohort study of 10,829 children
** $p < 0.001$
a leukemias only; b acute lymphocytic leukemia only; c acute nonlymphocytic leukemia only; d brain tumors only; e neuroblastoma only; f Wilms' tumor only.

Preconception Exposure to Ionizing Radiation

Of all occupational health issues, the one that possibly has received the most attention in the last three years is the suggestion that paternal preconception exposure to ionizing radiation increases the risk of childhood cancer.

In the February 17, 1990, issue of *British Medical Journal*, Dr. Martin Gardner and colleagues from the University of Southampton published an article on childhood leukemia.[11] They suggested that a cause for high leukemia rates observed at Sellafield, England, was the radiation doses that fathers of leukemia cases had received while working at the British Nuclear Fuels Limited facility. The interpretation was that the risk of leukemia was elevated in the offspring of nuclear workers because of genetic changes in germ cells (mutations) related to radiation exposure that may be leukemogenic.

In an attempt to identify the cause of a cluster of childhood cancers in the vicinity of the Sellafield nuclear plant in West Cumbria, Gardner et al.[11,12] conducted a case-control study of cases of leukemia and lymphoma. Examining a wide variety of risk factors, the authors demonstrated that relative risks for leukemia and non-Hodgkin's lymphoma were higher in children born near Sellafield and in children of fathers employed at the facility, particularly fathers with high radiation doses before conception.

The case-control study of Gardner et al.[11,12] determined all known cases of leukemia and lymphoma among residents of the West Cumbria Health Authority who were diagnosed between 1950 and 1985, were born in the area, and were younger than 25 at the time of diagnosis. The investigators attempted to select eight "area" controls and eight "local" controls for each case from the birth register where the case's birth was recorded, matched on sex and time of birth and whose mothers resided in West Cumbria at the time of the birth (area controls) or whose mothers resided in the same civil parish as the case (local controls). Some controls fell into both groups. Excluded were potential controls who had died or were not living in West Cumbria at the time cancer was diagnosed in the case to whom they were matched.

Evidence that paternal employment at Sellafield was associated with an increased risk of leukemia in the workers' children was established by linking fathers of cases and controls to the facility's employment and radiation records. Fathers of cases who had worked at Sellafield had accumulated higher preconception doses of external radiation than had fathers of controls. Fathers of four of 46 children with leukemia versus five of 288 controls had cumulative exposure levels above 100 mSv, for a relative risk of 6.2 (95% CI 1.5–26). In addition to the risk associated with cumulative doses above 100 mSv, there appeared to be an increased risk with doses above 10 mSv during the 6 months immediately before conception. Even if analyses are restricted to offspring of fathers who had been recorded as ever having had a "positive" external radiation dose, there is a marked difference in exposure histories between cases and controls.

The Gardner study and the context and implications of the findings are discussed extensively in a recent review.[52] Importantly, the associations reported by Gardner et al.[11] are not supported by findings in the offspring of men exposed to ionizing radiation at Hiroshima and Nagasaki. For example, Ishimaru, Ichimaru, and Mihami[25] reported that children of fathers exposed to a single high dose of radiation were not at increased risk for leukemia. Gardner et al.[11] briefly considered this aspect of their study and noted differences in dose rate, with the Japanese having acute high-dose exposures. Also, few conceptions occurred in the

TABLE 3. Parental Occupational Exposures to Metals and Risk of Childhood Cancer: Review of Studies

Reference	Number of Cases	Age (Years)	Incident/ Dead Cases	Source of Controls	Maternal/ Paternal Exposure	Time of Exposure	Type of Exposure Information	Findings	Potential Confounders Considered
All Cancers									
Olsen, de Nully Brown, Schulgen, & Jensen[42]	1,721	<15	I	Population register	M & P	At conception	Job title, company and industry in pension records	OR* = 2.2[†] for parental work in manufacture of iron and metal structures	Child's sex and date of birth and parental age
Feingold, Savitz, & John[8]	252	<15	I	Random-digit-dialing	M & P	Year prior to birth	Job title and industry from parental interview used in job-exposure matrix[20]	OR = 0.9–2.6 for paternal exposure to specific metals	Child's age and sex, telephone exchange, paternal education, maternal smoking
Leukemias and Lymphomas									
Buckley, Robison, Swotinsky, et al.[2]	178	<18	I[c]	Random-digit-dialing	M & P	From one year prior to pregnancy to one year prior to diagnosis	Occupations and exposures from parental interviews	OR = 1.0–∞ for paternal lead exposure (trend $p = 0.03$), highest risk after pregnancy; OR = 4.0–6.0 for maternal metal dust exposure (trend $p = 0.02$), highest risk with preconception exposure (OR = 5.5[†])	Child's date of birth and race
Feingold, Savitz, & John[8]	59	<15	I[b]	Random-digit-dialing	M & P	Year prior to birth	Job title and industry from parental interview used in job-exposure matrix[20]	OR = 0.7–1.7 for paternal exposure to specific metals	Child's age and sex, telephone exchange, paternal education, maternal smoking

Reference	No.	Age	Type	Source	Parent	Exposure period	Exposure assessment	Results	Matching/adjustment variables
Roman, Watson, Beral, et al.[46]	51	< 5	I	Hospital delivery registers and live birth registers	P	At birth and from 3 years before birth to diagnosis	Occupation on birth certificate and from parental interviews	OR = 1.1–1.5 for occupation in engineering and metals	Child's sex, date of birth, and area of residence at birth and diagnosis

Brain and Nervous System

Reference	No.	Age	Type	Source	Parent	Exposure period	Exposure assessment	Results	Matching/adjustment variables
Spitz & Johnson[55]	157	< 15	D^e	Birth certificates	P	At birth	Occupation and industry on birth certificate used in job-exposure clusters[23]	OR = 2.13–2.14† for cluster that includes welders (and electric and electronics workers)	Child's birth year
Wilkins & Koutras[63]	491	< 20	D^d	Birth certificates	P	At birth	Occupation and industry on birth certificate used in job-exposure matrix[20]	OR = 1.8† for employment in metal industry; OR = 2.6 for occupations in metal fabrication; OR = 2.7 for welders and cutters; OR = 5.0 for occupation in metal processing; OR = 1.1–1.6 for occupations in metal machinery and metal working	Child's age, race, sex, birth order and birthweight, parental age and proportion of farmland in county of residence
Wilkins & Sinks[66]	110	< 20	I^d	Random-digit-dialing	M & P	Preconception, prenatal, postnatal periods	Occupation and industry from parental interviews used in job-exposure matrix[20] and job-exposure clusters[23]	OR = 1.7–3.3† for paternal work in metal industry (highest risk for preconception); OR = 1.7–2.7† for parental exposures in clusters including metals (highest risk postnatal for fathers, preconception for mothers)	Child's year of birth, race, and sex

(Continued on next page)

TABLE 3. Parental Occupational Exposures to Metals and Risk of Childhood Cancer: Review of Studies (*Continued*)

Reference	Number of Cases	Age (Years)	Incident/ Dead Cases	Source of Controls	Maternal/ Paternal Exposure	Time of Exposure	Type of Exposure Information	Findings	Potential Confounders Considered
Feingold, Savitz, & John[8]	67	<15	I[d]	Random-digit-dialing	P	Year prior to birth	Job title and industry from parental interview used in job-exposure matrix[20]	OR = 0.8–2.1 for specific metal exposures	Child's age and sex, telephone exchange, paternal education, maternal smoking
Kuijten, Bunin, Nass, Meadows[32]	163	<15	I[d]	Random-digit-dialing	M & P	Preconception, prenatal, and postnatal periods	Job title and industry from parental interviews	OR = 0.8–1.1 for paternal metal occupations	Child's age, race and telephone area code
Urinary Tract Cancers									
Wilkins & Sinks,[64]	62	All	I[f]	Birth certificates	P	At birth	Occupation and industry on birth certificate used for job-exposure matrix[20]	OR = 0.22–0.38 for work in metal industry; OR = 0.7–1.3 for exposure to lead compounds; OR = 1.1 for exposure to nickel or cadmium compounds; OR = 4.0 for exposure to calcium or mercury	Child's age, sex and race and maternal county of residence
Wilson & Sinks[65]	62	All	I[f]	Birth certificates	P	At birth	Occupation on child's birth certificate	OR = 1.25 for lead-related occupations	Child's race, sex, and year of birth and maternal county of residence
Bunin, Nass, Kramer, & Meadows[4]	88 (whites only)	<15	I[f]	Random-digit-dialing	M & P	Preconception, prenatal, and birth to six months before diagnosis	Job and industry from prenatal interviews used in job-exposure matrix[20] and job-exposure clusters[23]	OR = 1.6–6.0 for paternal exposure in clusters including metals (highest risk for genetic cases exposed in preconception or prenatal period)	Child's race and date of birth and telephone area code and prefix and proxy interview

Reference	No.	Age	Case ascertainment		Source	Parent	Exposure period	Exposure assessment	Results	Adjustment/matching factors
Olsen, de Nully Brown, Schulgen, & Jensen[42]	132	<15	I[f]		Population register	M & P	At conception	Job title company and industry in pension fund records	OR = 7.1[†] for paternal work in manufacture of iron and metal structures	Child's sex and date of birth, parental age
Retinoblastoma										
Bunin, Petrakova, Meadows, et al.[5]	201	All	I		Random-digit-dialing	M & P	Preconception, postconception	Occupation from parental interviews used in job exposure matrix[20] and job-exposure clusters[23]	OR = 1.3–∞[†] for paternal work in metal manufacturing (risk highest in sporadic cases); OR = 1.7–5.0[†] for paternal welders and machinists (risk highest in nonheritable cases); OR = 0.9–3.3[†] for paternal metal-related occupations (risk highest in nonheritable cases)	Child's date of birth, race and telephone area code and first five digits of phone number
Hepatoblastoma										
Buckley, Sather, Ruccione, et al.[3]	75	All	I		Random-digit-dialing	M & P	Ever	Occupations and exposures from parental interviews	OR = 7.0[†]–∞ for maternal occupation in metals, welding, or soldering; OR = 8.0[†] for all combined (highest risk for preconception and prenatal period); OR = 0.9–1.0 for paternal welding or soldering; OR = 3.0 for paternal occupation in metals; OR = 2.6[†] for either parent exposed to metals	Child's age, other chemical exposures

* OR = odds ratio.
† $p < 0.05$
** $p < 0.001$
†† cohort study of 10,829 children.
a leukemias only; b acute lymphocytic leukemia only; c acute nonlymphocytic leukemia only; d brain tumors only; e neuroblastoma only; f Wilms' tumor only.

TABLE 4. Parental Textile-related Occupations and Risk of Childhood Cancer: Review of Studies

Reference	Number of Cases	Age (Years)	Incident/Dead Cases	Source of Controls	Maternal/Paternal Exposure	Time of Exposure	Type of Exposure Information	Findings	Potential Confounders Considered
All Cancers									
Fabia & Thuy[7]	386	< 5	D	Birth certificates	P	At birth	Occupation on child's birth certificate	OR* = 2.02[†] for tailor, weaver, furrier	Parental age, residency, child's birth-date
Sanders, White, & Draper[47]	2,771	< 15	D[a]	Childhood deaths	P	At child's death	Occupation on child's death certificate	PMR* = 60–94 for textile or clothing workers	Social class
Leukemias and Lymphomas									
Van Steensel-Moll, Valkenburg, & Van Zanen[59]	519	< 15	I[b]	Same census region as case	M & P	During pregnancy, one year before diagnosis	Occupation from parental interviews	OR = 4.7[†] for maternal work in textile industry during pregnancy	Child's date of birth and sex, place of residence at diagnosis, birth order, father's education
Lowengart, Peters, Cicioni, et al.[34]	123	< 11	I[a]	Friends of case or random-digit-dialing	M & P	One year pre-conception to one year prediagnosis	Occupations and exposures from maternal interviews	OR = 1.4 for paternal textile occupation	Child's age, sex, race and Hispanic origin and socio-economic status

Reference	No.	Age	Type	Source of Cases	Parent	Timing	Exposure Assessment	Results	Adjustment
Magnani, Pastore, Luzzatto, & Terracini[36]	183	All	I	Hospitalized children, excluding cancer, Down's syndrome, β-thalassemia, infections, mononucleosis, lymphadenitis, or unexplained splenic enlargement	M & P	Up to child's birth and between birth and diagnosis	Occupations from interviews with closest relatives	OR = 10.1[†c] for maternal textile spinner and winder; OR = 1.9–4.3[†c] for maternal work in textile industry; OR = 10.1[†c] for paternal textile worker associated with acute nonlymphocytic leukemia; OR = 6.0[†c]–7.6[†c] for paternal work in textile industry	Socioeconomic status
Infante-Rivard, Mur, Armstrong, et al.[24]	128	<15	I[b]	Census	M	During pregnancy	Occupation and exposures from maternal interviews	OR = 5.5[†] for maternal exposure to dusts: cotton, wool, synthetic fibers	Child's year of birth, sex and municipality at diagnosis
Brain and Nervous System									
Spitz & Johnson[55]	157	<15	D[e]	Birth certificates	P	At birth	Occupation and industry on birth certificate used in job-exposure clusters[23]	OR = 16.74 for exposure to dusts	Child's birth year
Wilkins & Koutras[63]	491	<20	D[d]	Birth certificates	P	At birth	Industry and occupation on birth certificate used in job-exposure matrix[20]	OR = 1.9 for work in textiles	Child's age, race sex, birth order and birthweight, parental age, and proportion of farmland in county of residence

(Continued on next page)

TABLE 4. Parental Textile-related Occupations and Risk of Childhood Cancer: Review of Studies *(Continued)*

Reference	Number of Cases	Age (Years)	Incident/ Dead Cases	Source of Controls	Maternal/ Paternal Exposure	Time of Exposure	Type of Exposure Information	Findings	Potential Confounders Considered
Wilkins & Sinks[66]	110	<20	I[d]	Random-digit-dialing	M & P	Preconception, prenatal, and postnatal periods	Occupation and industry from parental interviews used in job-exposure matrix[20] and job-exposure cluster[23]	OR = 0.3 for maternal work in textiles	Child's year of birth, race, and sex
Olsen, de Nully Brown, Schulgen, & Jensen[42]	416	<15	I	Population register	M & P	At conception	Job title, company and industry in pension fund records	OR = 2.2[†] for maternal work in textile industry	Child's sex and date of birth, parental age
Urinary Tract Cancers									
Wilkins & Sinks[64]	62	All	I[f]	Birth certificates	P	At birth	Occupation and industry on birth certificate used for job-exposure matrix[20]	OR = 1.0 for work in textiles	Child's age, sex and race and maternal county of residence
Soft Tissue Sarcomas									
Magnani, Pastore, Luzzatto, et al.[35]	88	All	I	Hospitalized children without cancer, Down's syndrome, β-thalassemia, infections, mononucleosis, lymphadenitis, or unspecified splenic enlargement	M & P	Before birth, and birth to diagnosis	Occupations from interviews with close relatives	OR = 4.3[†] for maternal home textile work up to child's birth; OR = 7.0[†] for paternal textile and garment work up to child's birth; OR = 4.0[†] for maternal spinning and weaving up to child's birth; OR = 14.2 for maternal weaver birth to diagnosis	Clinical center

* Abbreviations: OR = odds ratio; PMR = proportionate mortality ratio.
† $p < 0.05$
** $p < 0.001$
†† cohort study of 10,829 children
a leukemias only; b acute lymphocytic leukemia only; c acute nonlymphocytic leukemia only; d brain tumors only; e neuroblastoma only; f Wilms' tumor only.

period shortly after the bombings, which is when paternal effects might be most likely to occur. In addition to human data, experimental animal data also suggested an effect of paternal radiation exposure on subsequent cancer risks in offspring.[40]

McKinney et al.[37] examined the parental occupations of children with leukemia and non-Hodgkin's lymphoma in West Cumbria, North Humberside, and Gateshead. The analysis included 109 cases and 206 controls matched to the cases on the basis of date of birth, sex, and health district. Data were collected by interview and included information on both ionizing and nonionizing radiation exposure. Significant associations were demonstrated for paternal preconceptional, periconceptional/gestational, and postnatal radiation exposures, but not for work in the nuclear industry. No dosimetric data were presented. There is some overlap in cases between this study and Gardner et al.,[11] but the data for this study were collected before the results of the Gardner study were published. This should reduce the possibility of recall bias influencing the results.

Urquhart et al.[58] conducted a case-control study of childhood leukemia and non-Hodgkin's lymphoma cases in the vicinity of Dounreay nuclear installation in Scotland. Analyses were based on 13 cases diagnosed before age 15 and 55 controls matched on sex, date of birth, and mother's area of residence at the time of the case's birth. Paternal occupation was determined, and fathers were matched with nuclear worker registries to determine radiation doses. No significant associations were found between cancer risk and father's lifetime preconceptional radiation dose. No increased risk was observed if the father's lifetime radiation dose prior to conception was more than 100 mSv or if the dose in the six months prior to conception was more than 10 mSv.

In a comment on the Dounreay study, Gardner[10] noted the Dounreay doses are smaller than the Sellafield doses and that the number of Dounreay cases was small. He concluded that the results of the Dounreay study[58] are not inconsistent with the findings of the Sellafield study.[11]

Kinlen, Clarke, and Balkwill[30] conducted a case-control study of cases of leukemia and non-Hodgkin's lymphoma diagnosed in Scotland. Participants were younger than 25 and born in or after 1958. The investigators included relevant cases from North Cumbria in England since workers at one Scottish nuclear site live across the border in that area. For cases born in Scotland, three controls were selected from births of the same sex occurring in the same county. The names of fathers of cases and controls were matched against files of nuclear workers. Information was obtained on radiation doses for men who were employed in the nuclear industry. No significantly increased cancer risk was associated with preconceptional radiation exposure.

Sorahan and Roberts[54] examined cases of childhood cancers from the Oxford Survey of Childhood Cancers for potential associations between paternal occupational exposure to ionizing radiation and cancer risks. Cases of all types of childhood cancers were included. To provide an independent test of the findings of Gardner et al.,[11] cases whose fathers were Sellafield employees were excluded. Exposure was estimated based on occupational history. Doses for external radiation were estimated and grouped according to the exposure groupings used by Gardner et al.[11] Potential for exposure to radionuclides also was estimated. There were no significantly elevated relative risks associated with increasing estimated doses of external radiation. For radionuclide exposure, the relative risk for all childhood cancers was 2.70 (95% CI 1.31–5.58), but the risks for leukemia and non-Hodgkin's lymphoma were not elevated.

TABLE 5. Parental Exposures to Wood, Paper and Pulp and Risk of Childhood Cancer: Review of Studies

Reference	Number of Cases	Age (Years)	Incident/ Dead Cases	Source of Controls	Maternal/ Paternal Exposure	Time of Exposure	Type of Exposure Information	Findings	Potential Confounders Considered
All Cancers									
Fabia & Thuy[7]	386	< 5	D	Birth certificates	P	At birth	Occupation on child's birth certificate	NSA* with lumberman or construction workers	Parental age and residence, child's birthdate
Sanders, White, & Draper[47]	6,920	< 15	D	Childhood deaths	P	At child's death	Occupation on child's death certificate	PMR* = 94–100 for woodworkers or construction workers; PMR = 99–119 for paper workers	Social class
Leukemias and Lymphomas									
Buckley, Robison, Swotinsky, et al.[2]	178	< 18	I^c	Random-digit-dialing	M & P	One year preconception to one year prediagnosis	Occupations and exposures from parental interviews	OR = 0–∞ for maternal exposure to sawdust (trend $p = 0.03$), highest risk for exposure before pregnancy	Child's date of birth and race
Magnani, Pastore, Luzzatto, & Terracini[36]	183	All	I	Hospitalized children without cancer, Down's syndrome, β-thalassemia, infections, mononucleosis, lymphadenitis, or unspecified splenic enlargement	M & P	Anytime before birth, and birth to diagnosis	Occupations from interviews with closest relative	OR = 2.1–7.1† for paternal work with wood and furniture or work in building industry associated with acute lymphocytic leukemia; OR = 6.6 for paternal carpenter after birth; OR = 10.1–12.1† for paternal construction worker	Socioeconomic status
Olsen, de Nully Brown, Schulgen, & Jensen[42]	603	< 15	I	Population register	M & P	At conception	Job title, company and industry in pension records	OR = 3.1† for maternal work in construction	Child's sex and date of birth, parental age

Author	No.	Age	Design	Source		Timing	Exposure assessment	Results	Variables controlled
Roman, Watson, Beral, et al.[46]	51	< 5	I	Hospital delivery registers and live birth registers	P	At birth and from 3 years before birth to diagnosis	Occupation on birth certificate and from parental interviews	OR = 0.6–1.4 for occupation in wood	Child's sex, date of birth and area of residence at birth and diagnosis
Brain and Nervous System Tumors									
Spitz & Johnson[55]	157	< 15	D^e	Birth certificates	P	At birth	Occupation and industry on birth certificate used in job-exposure clusters[23]	OR = 0.87 for work in construction industry	Child's birth year
Johnson, Annegers, Frankowski, et al.[26]	499	< 15	D	Birth certificates	P	At birth	Occupation and industry on child's birth certificate	OR = 4.0 for paper and pulp mill workers; OR = 2.7 for workers in paper, pulp mill and paper products industries	Child's birthdate, race and sex
Nasca, Baptiste, MacCubbin, et al.[39]	338	< 15	I	Birth certificates	P	At birth, at diagnosis	Occupation and industry from maternal interviews	OR = 1.62 for work in pulp and paper industry at birth; OR = 2.09 for work in pulp and paper industry at diagnosis	Child's age, sex and race
Wilkins & Koutras[63]	491	< 20	D^d	Birth certificate	P	At birth	Industry and occupation on birth certificate used in job-exposure matrix[20]	OR = 2.3† for work in construction; OR = 1.9 for carpenters; OR = 0.9 for work in paper and wood occupations	Child's age, race, sex, birth order, and birth-weight, parental age and proportion of farmland in county of residence

(Continued on next page)

TABLE 5. Parental Exposures to Wood, Paper and Pulp and Risk of Childhood Cancer: Review of Studies (*Continued*)

Reference	Number of Cases	Age (Years)	Incident/ Dead Cases	Source of Controls	Maternal/ Paternal Exposure	Time of Exposure	Type of Exposure Information	Findings	Potential Confounders Considered
Wilkins & Sinks[66]	110	<20	I[d]	Random-digit-dialing	M & P	Preconception, prenatal, and postnatal periods	Occupation and industry from parental interviews used in job-exposure matrix[20] and job-exposure clusters[23]	OR = 0.9–1.8 for paternal work in construction industry; OR = 1.4–∞ for paternal work in paper and wood industry	Child's year of birth, race and sex
Olsen, de Nully Brown, Schulgen, & Jensen[42]	416	<15	I	Population register	M & P	At conception	Job title, company and industry from pension fund records	OR = 2.3[†] for paternal work in carpentry	Child's sex and date of birth, parental age
Kuijten, Bunin, Nass, & Meadows[32]	163	<15	I[d]	Random-digit-dialing	M & P	Preconception, prenatal, and postnatal periods	Job title and industry from parental interviews	OR = 2.0–∞ for paternal work in paper and pulp mill industry; OR = 0.8–1.1 for paternal work in construction	Child's age, race and telephone area code
Urinary Tract Cancers									
Wilkins & Sinks[64]	62	All	I[f]	Birth certificates	P	At birth	Occupation and industry on birth certificate used in job-exposure matrix[20]	OR = 0.66–1.0 for work in paper and wood industry	Child's age, sex and race and maternal county of residence

Wilkins & Sinks[65]	62	All	I[f]	Birth certificate	P	At birth	Occupation on child's birth certificate	OR = 1.0 for lumberman	Child's race, sex and year of birth and maternal county of residence
Olsen, de Nully Brown, Schulgen, & Jensen[42]	132	< 15	I[f]	Population register	M & P	At conception	Job title, company and industry in pension fund records	OR = 2.9[†] for paternal work in wood and furniture industry	Child's sex and date of birth, parental age
Soft Tissue Sarcoma									
Magnani, Pastore, Luzzatto, et al.[35]	88	All	I	Hospitalized children without cancer, Down's syndrome, β-thalassemia, infections, mononucleosis, lymphadenitis, or unspecified splenic enlargement	M & P	Before birth, and birth to diagnosis	Occupations from interviews with close relatives	OR = 2.7[†] for paternal building worker from birth to diagnosis	Clinical center

* Abbreviations: OR = odds ratio; PMR = proportionate mortality ratio.
† p < 0.05   ** p < 0.001   †† cohort study of 10,829 children
a leukemias only; b acute lymphocytic leukemia only; c acute nonlymphocytic leukemia only; d brain tumors only; e neuroblastoma only; f Wilms' tumor only.

In August 1992, the Atomic Energy Control Board of Canada reported results of a case-control study of fathers' occupational ionizing radiation exposure and childhood leukemia in Ontario, Canada.[38] The study was conducted using leukemia cases in the vicinities of five nuclear facilities in Ontario and was designed to test the hypothesis growing out of the Sellafield study that linked paternal radiation exposure and childhood leukemia risk. It included 112 cases, who were younger than 15 at diagnosis between 1950 and 1988 and who were born to women who resided in the vicinity of an operating nuclear facility. Eight birth certificate controls were matched to each case by date of birth and mother's residence at birth (n = 890 matched controls).

Fathers of the subjects were linked to occupational radiation records of the Canadian National Dose Registry (NDR). Missing names, initials, and birth date led to problems with linkage. Computer exposure histories were obtained from NDR records. Information on whole body dose and internal dose was obtained for lifetime and annual doses.

Covariables examined included maternal age, birthweight, birth order, and sex. There was also an indicator of distance between a child's residence at birth (center of census subdivision) and the nearest nuclear facility.

Analyses included whole body dose, tritium dose and radon exposures during three preconception periods: lifetime, 6 months, and 3 months prior to conception. The findings reported by McLaughlin et al.[38] do not support the hypothesis that childhood leukemia is associated with paternal preconception occupational ionizing radiation exposure.

Roman et al.[46] recently reported the results of a study of leukemia and non-Hodgkin's lymphoma in children younger than age 5 from the West Berkshire and Basingstoke and North Hampshire District Health Authorities. The children had to have been born and diagnosed in the study area. There were 54 cases and six controls for each case, for a total of 324 controls. Data were collected from the child's birth certificate, personal interview of the parents, mother's obstetric notes, and employment and health physics notes held by the nuclear industry. Parents' names and dates of birth were linked to employment and health physics records of the Atomic Weapons Establishment, the Atomic Energy Authority, and the National Registry of Radiation Workers.

The risk of leukemia or non-Hodgkin's lymphoma was significantly increased in children whose fathers had been monitored for exposure to ionizing radiation because they worked in areas where exposure to ionizing radiation was possible. Importantly, none of the fathers had been monitored for exposure at around the time of their child's conception or in the 4 years preceding that date. In addition, the recorded doses were low, with no fathers receiving cumulative whole body doses above 5 mSv.

Roman et al.[46] interpret their data as suggesting that the children of men who are monitored for external radiation might be at increased risk of leukemia. They do not believe that association with exposure to external penetrating radiation is likely to be the explanation. They suggest that a more plausible explanation is that exposure to external radiation is a marker of exposure to some other hazard, such as internal contamination with a chemical or radioactive substance. This is compatible with the findings from the Oxford Survey of Childhood Cancers[54] of an association between childhood cancer risk and paternal exposure to radionuclides but not to exposure to external radiation. It might also help to explain the lack of consistency among studies regarding leukemia risk and radiation exposure, since it is possible that exposure to external radiation is not a relevant marker of exposure to other hazards in all the studies.[46] As Roman et al.[46] note, "The possibility that the effects could be due to internal contamination by radioactive substances, a chemical, or some other exposure at work should be explored."

Currently, one of the authors (LS) is conducting a case-control study of childhood cancers and paternal occupational exposure to ionizing radiation. The study includes leukemia, non-Hodgkin's lymphoma, and central nervous system cancers in children younger than age 15 at the time of diagnosis. Cases are being accumulated using multiple sources from the residents around the Department of Energy (DOE) Hanford Nuclear Facility in Washington state. The feasibility of expanding the study to include cases from around three additional DOE sites— Idaho National Engineering Laboratory, Oak Ridge National Laboratory, and the Savannah River Site—is being evaluated.

The design of the study is based on selection of matched controls from birth certificates. All data will be collected from existing record sources, including birth and death certificates, medical records, worker rosters, and dosimetry records. Names of cases' parents will be linked to rosters of workers at the nuclear facilities. For cases with a parent(s) employed at the facility, radiation exposure prior to conception will be determined along with information on other potentially hazardous exposures. Analyses will include the evaluation of radiation dose as a continuous variable, as well as odds ratios for dose categories similar to the dose categories used by Gardner et al.[11] and McLaughlin et al.[38]

Paternal Exposure to Electromagnetic Fields

During the last decade there has been growing concern regarding the potential effects on human health, including reproductive effects and carcinogenic potential in children, of nonionizing radiation, particularly extremely low frequency electromagnetic fields (EMF). Much of this concern arose out of earlier community studies of residential and household exposures.[9,50,51,57,61] While many of the issues involved are outside the scope of this discussion, one topic of relevance is associations between paternal exposure to EMF and subsequent risk of cancer in children. Several associations have been suggested between cancer risk and employment in "electrical occupations." Importantly, to our knowledge, all of the studies examining specific associations with electrical occupations have been restricted to father's occupation. NIOSH is considering studies of maternal occupational exposure to EMF and childhood cancer as a priority area.

The initial study of paternal occupational EMF exposure and childhood cancers was a study of neuroblastoma carried out in Texas.[55] Cases were identified from death certificates, and paternal occupation was determined using birth certificates. Controls were selected from birth certificates. In their examination of a number of occupational groupings, the authors identified statistically significant elevated odds ratios for electronics workers (OR 11.75 95% CI 1.40–98.55) and for a group of electrical occupations (OR 2.13 95% CI 1.05–4.35). Two subsequent case-control studies designed specifically to test the association between electrical occupations and neuroblastoma risk did not demonstrate statistically significant elevated risks,[5,62] but both found odds ratios above one for some combinations of electrical occupations.

Studies of childhood central nervous system (CNS) tumor also have examined associations with paternal employment in electrical occupations. In New York state, Nasca et al.[39] examined paternal occupation at birth and at diagnosis for a series of 338 cases of CNS cancers from the New York Cancer Registry. They observed elevated odds ratios, which were higher for the exposures at birth than at diagnosis, for two different groupings of electrical occupations, but these were not statistically significant.

In Texas, Johnson and Spitz[27] examined the relationship of deaths from CNS cancers among children and paternal occupations obtained from birth certificates. They found elevated odds ratios for several electrical occupational categories, but only for electricians (and construction electricians as a subcategory) was the odds ratio significantly elevated.

In summary, there are suggestive data for increased risks of two categories of childhood cancers, neuroblastomas and CNS tumors, associated with electrical occupations. Since EMF is not known to be mutagenic, there is no clear potential mechanism by which to relate preconception paternal EMF exposures to childhood cancer risk. It is possible that the occupations share an exposure other than to EMF, but the occupations are really quite heterogeneous. While Hatch[16] suggests that electrical occupations are not strongly correlated with other carcinogens, Johnson and Spitz[27] note that other relevant potential exposures may occur for electrical and electronic apparatus workers and workers in the electronics industry.

CONCLUSION

Evidence is increasing that childhood cancers should be considered as part of the array of occupational reproductive hazards. The studies we have reviewed have been based largely on the use of job titles or occupation as a surrogate for exposure. Thus, there is a clear need for improving exposure assessment methods. Issues of retrospective exposure assessment in epidemiologic studies are receiving increasing attention,[18] and much of this discussion is relevant to studies of parental exposures and childhood cancer risks.

Other important issues revolve around pathogenetic mechanisms and the timing of exposure. Preconception exposure of either parent could lead to genetic alterations that are transmitted to the offspring. This is the mechanism suggested for the association between paternal radiation exposure and childhood leukemia risk.[11] Exposures during gestation or early childhood could involve mechanisms for carcinogens similar to those proposed for adult cancers, and there is clear evidence for human transplacental carcinogenesis. A paternal contribution to cancer initiated during gestation could occur by transmission of carcinogenic agents through seminal fluid or through contaminated clothing, leading to maternal-fetal exposure. This latter mechanism could also result in chemical exposures during childhood.

Questions about the relevant timing of parental exposures are specific to the agents involved. For example, paternal exposures at different points in the cycle of spermatogenesis have different potential effects. For both maternal and paternal chemical exposures, differences between substances in the pharmacokinetics , excretion, and storage are important. For example, the time between exposure to solvents and the effect on an embryo is relatively brief, but lead could be released from tissue stores for an extended time following exposure. The complex interplay among exposure, dose, biologically effective dose, pathogenesis, and latency requires a considerable amount of additional attention.

In conclusion, evidence suggests that some childhood cancers could be related to parental occupational exposures to chemical and physical agents. To understand the true significance of the associations that have been demonstrated requires refinement of study methods and increased emphasis on understanding exposure and dose and the biological mechanisms of carcinogenesis.

REFERENCES

1. Bleyer WA: What can be learned about childhood cancer from "Cancer Statistics Review 1973–1988." Cancer 71(suppl):3229–3236, 1993.
2. Buckley JD, Robison LL, Swotinsky R, et al: Occupational exposures of parents of children with acute nonlymphocytic leukemia: A report from the Children's Cancer Study Group. Cancer Res 49:4030–4037, 1989.
3. Buckley JD, Sather H, Ruccione K, et al: Case-control study of risk factors for hepatoblastoma: A report from the Children's Cancer Study Group. Cancer 64:1169–1176, 1989.
4. Bunin GR, Nass CC, Kramer S, Meadows AT: Parental occupation and Wilms' tumor: Results of a case-control study. Cancer Res 49:725–729, 1989.
5. Bunin GR, Petrakova A, Meadows AT, et al: Occupations of parents of children with retino-blastoma: A report from the Children's Cancer Study Group. Cancer Res 50:7129–7133, 1990.
6. Bunin GR, Ward E, Kramer S, et al: Neuroblastoma and parental occupation. Am J Epidemiol 131:776–780, 1990.
7. Fabia J, Thuy TD: Occupation of father at time of birth of children dying of malignant disease. Br J Prev Soc Med 28:98–100, 1974.
8. Feingold L, Savitz DA, John EM: Use of a job-exposure matrix to evaluate parental occupation and childhood cancer. Cancer Causes Control 3:161–169, 1992.
9. Fulton JP, Cobb S, Preble L, et al: Electrical wiring configurations and childhood leukemia in Rhode Island. Am J Epidemiol 111:292–296, 1980.
10. Gardner MJ: Radiation workers and childhood leukemia. BMJ 302:907, 1991.
11. Gardner MJ, Snee MP, Hall AJ, et al: Results of case-control study of leukaemia and lymphoma among young people near Sellafield nuclear plant in West Cumbria. BMJ 300:423–429, 1990.
12. Gardner MJ, Hall AJ, Snee MP, et al: Methods and basic data of case-control study of leukaemia and lymphoma among young people near Sellafield nuclear plant in West Cumbria. BMJ 300:429–434, 1990.
13. Gold EB, Leviton A, Lopez R, et al: Parental smoking and risk of childhood brain tumors. Am J Epidemiol 137:620–628, 1993.
14. Gold EB, Diener MD, Szklo M: Parental occupations and cancer in children: A case-control study and review of the methodologic issues. J Occup Med 24:578–584, 1982.
15. Hakulinen T, Salonen T, Teppo L: Cancer in the offspring of fathers in hydrocarbon-related occupations. Br J Prev Soc Med 30:138–140, 1976.
16. Hatch M: The epidemiology of electric and magnetic field exposures in the power frequency range and reproductive outcomes. Paediatr Perinat Epidemiol 6:198–214, 1992.
17. Hemminki K, Saloniemi I, Salonen T: Childhood cancer and parental occupation in Finland. J Epidemiol Community Health 35:11–15, 1981.
18. Herrick RF, Stewart PA: International workshop on retrospective exposure assessment for occupational epidemiologic studies. Appl Occup Environ Hyg 6:417–420, 1991.
19. Hicks N, Zack M, Caldwell GG, et al: Childhood cancer and occupational radiation exposure in parents. Cancer 53:1637–1643, 1984.
20. Hoar SK, Morrison AS, Cole P, et al: An occupation and exposure linkage system for the study of occupational carcinogenesis. J Occup Med 22:722–726, 1980.
21. Holly EA, Aston DA, Ahn DK, Kristiansen JJ: Ewing's bone sarcoma, paternal occupational exposure and other factors. Am J Epidemiol 135:122–129, 1992.
22. Howe GR, Burch JD, Chiarelli AM, et al: An exploratory case-control study of brain tumors in children. Cancer Res 49:4349–4352, 1989.
23. Hsieh CC, Walker AM, Hoar SK: Grouping occupations according to carcinogenic potential: Occupation clusters from an exposure linkage system. Am J Epidemiol 117:575–589, 1983.
24. Infante-Rivard C, Mur P, Armstrong B, et al: Acute lymphoblastic leukaemia among Spanish children and mothers' occupation: A case-control study. J Epidemiol Community Health 45:11–15, 1991.
25. Ishimaru T, Ichimaru M, Mikami M: Leukemia incidence among individuals exposed in utero, children of atomic bomb survivors and their controls, Hiroshima and Nagasaki, 1945–1979. Hiroshima, Radiation Effects Research Foundation, 1981, RERF Technical Report 11–81.

26. Johnson CC, Annegers JF, Frankowski RF, et al: Childhood nervous system tumors—an evaluation of the association with paternal occupational exposure to hydrocarbons. Am J Epidemiol 126:605–613, 1987.
27. Johnson C, Spitz M: Childhood nervous system tumors: An assessment of risk associated with paternal occupations involving use, repair or manufacture of electrical and electronic equipment. Int J Epidemiol 18:756–762, 1989.
28. Johnston HE, Mann JR, Williams J, et al: The inter-regional, epidemiological study of childhood cancer (IRESCC): Case-control study in children with germ cell tumours. Carcinogenesis 7:717–722, 1986.
29. Kantor AF, Curnen MGM, Meigs JW, et al: Occupation of fathers of patients with Wilms' tumor. J Epidemiol Community Health 33:253–256, 1979.
30. Kinlen LJ, Clark K, Balkwill A: Paternal preconceptional radiation exposure in the nuclear industry and leukaemia and non-Hodgkin's lymphoma in young people in Scotland. BMJ 306:1153–1158, 1993.
31. Kristensen P, Andersen A: A cohort study on cancer incidence in offspring of male printing workers. Epidemiology 3:6–10, 1992.
32. Kuitjen RR, Bunin GR, Nass CC, Meadows AT: Parental occupation and childhood astrocytoma: Results of a case-control study. Cancer Res 52:782–786, 1992.
33. Kwa SL, Fine LJ: The association between parental occupation and childhood malignancy. J Occup Med 22:792–794, 1980.
34. Lowengart RA, Peters JM, Cicioni C, et al: An epidemiologic case-control study of central nervous system tumors in children and parental occupational exposures. Am J Epidemiol 128:1256–1265, 1988.
35. Magnani C, Pastore G, Luzzatto L, et al: Risk factors for soft tissue sarcomas in childhood: A case-control study. Tumori 75:396–400, 1989.
36. Magnani C, Pastore G, Luzzatto L, Terracini B: Parental occupation and other environmental factors in the etiology of leukemias and non-Hodgkin's lymphomas in childhood: A case-control study. Tumori 76:413–419, 1990.
37. McKinney PA, Alexander FE, Cartwright RA, Parker L: Parental occupations of children with leukaemia in west Cumbria, north Humberside, and Gateshead. BMJ 302:681–687, 1991.
38. McLaughlin JR, King WD, Anderson TW, et al: Paternal radiation exposure and leukaemia in offspring: The Ontario case-control study. BMJ 307:959–966, 1993.
39. Nasca PC, Baptiste MS, MacCubbin PA, et al: An epidemiologic case-control study of cental nervous system tumors in children and parental occupational exposures. Am J Epidemiol 128:1256–1265, 1988.
40. Nomura T: Parental exposure to X rays and chemicals induces heritable tumours and anomalies in mice. Nature 296:575–577, 1982.
41. O'Leary LM, Hicks AM, Peters JM, London S: Parental occupational exposures and risk of childhood cancer: A review. Am J Ind Med 20:17–35, 1991.
42. Olsen JH, de Nully Brown P, Schulgen G, Jensen OM: Parental employment at time of conception and risk of cancer in offpsring. Eur J Cancer 27:958–965, 1991.
43. Olshan AF, Breslow NE, Daling JR, et al: Childhood brain tumors and paternal occupation in the aerospace industry. J Natl Cancer Inst 77:17–19, 1986.
44. Olshan AF, Faustman EM: Male-mediated developmental toxicity. Reprod Toxicol 7:191–202, 1993.
45. Peters JM, Preston-Martin S, Yu MC: Brain tumors in children and occupational exposure of parents. Science 213:235–237, 1981.
46. Roman E, Watson A, Beral V, et al: Case-control study of leukaemia and non-Hodgkin's lymphoma among children aged 0–4 years living in West Berkshire and North Hampshire health districts. BMJ 306:615–621, 1993.
47. Sanders BM, White GC, Draper GJ: Occupations of fathers of children dying from neoplasms. J Epidemiol Community Health 35:245–250, 1981.
48. Savitz DA: Childhood cancer. Occup Med State Art Rev 1:415–429, 1981.
49. Savitz DA, Chen J: Parental occupations and childhood cancer: Review of epidemiologic studies. Environ Health Perspect 88:325–337, 1990.
50. Savitz DA, Wachtel H, Barnes FA, et al: Case-control study of childhood cancer and exposure to 60 MHz magnetic fields. Am J Epidemiol 128:21–28, 1988.
51. Savitz DA, John EM, Kleckner RC: Magnetic field exposure from electric appliances and childhood cancer. Am J Epidemiol 131:763–773, 1990.
52. Sever LE: Parental radiation exposure and children's health: Are there effects on the second generation? Occup Med 6:613–627, 1991.
53. Shaw GM, Lavey R, Jackson R, et al: Association of childhood leukemia with maternal age, birth

order and paternal occupation. Am J Epidemiol 119:788–795, 1984.

54. Sorahan T, Roberts PJ: Childhood cancer and paternal exposure to ionizing radiation: Preliminary findings from the Oxford Survey of Childhood Cancers. Am J Ind Med 23:343–354, 1993.
55. Spitz M, Johnson C: Neuroblastoma and paternal occupation: A case-control analysis. Am J Epidemiol 121:924–929, 1985.
56. Terracini B, Pastore G, Segnan N: Association of father's occupation and cancer in children. Biol Res Preg Perinatol 4:40–45, 1983.
57. Tomenius L: 50 Hz electromagnetic environment and the incidence of childhood tumors in Stockholm County. Bioelectromagnetics 7:191–207, 1986.
58. Urquhart JD, Black RJ, Muirhead MJ, et al: Case-control study of leukaemia and non–Hodgkin's lymphoma in children in Caithness near the Dounreay nuclear installation. BMJ 302:687–692, 1991.
59. Van Steensel-Moll HA, Valkenburg HA, Van Zanen GE: Childhood leukemia and parental occupation: A register-based case-control study. Am J Epidemiol 121:216–224, 1985.
60. Vianna NH, Kovasznay B, Polan A, et al: Infant leukemia and paternal exposure to motor vehicle exhaust fumes. J Occup Med 26:679–682, 1984.
61. Wertheimer N, Leeper E: Electrical wiring configurations and childhood cancer. Am J Epidemiol 109:273–284, 1979.
62. Wilkins JR, Hundley VD: Paternal occupational exposure to electromagnetic fields and neuroblastoma in offspring. Am J Epidemiol 131:995–1007, 1990.
63. Wilkins JR, Koutras RA: Paternal occupation and brain cancer in offspring: A mortality-based case-control study. Am J Ind Med 14:299–318, 1988.
64. Wilkins JR III, Sinks TH Jr: Occupational exposures among fathers of children with Wilms' tumor. J Occup Med 26:427–435, 1984.
65. Wilkins JR III, Sinks TH Jr: Paternal occupation and Wilms' tumour in offspring. J Epidemiol Community Health 38:7–11, 1984.
66. Wilkins JR III, Sinks TH: Parental occupation and intracranial neoplasms of childhood: Results of a case-control interview study. Am J Epidemiol 132:275–292, 1990.
67. Zack M, Cannon S, Loyd D, et al: Cancer in children of parents exposed to hydrocarbon-related industries and occupations. Am J Epidemiol 111:329–336, 1980.

CATHY L. SAIKI, MS
ELLEN B. GOLD, PhD
MARC B. SCHENKER, MD, MPH

WORKPLACE POLICY ON HAZARDS TO REPRODUCTIVE HEALTH

From the Division of Occupational/
Environmental Medicine and
Epidemiology
School of Medicine
and Institute of Toxicology
and Environmental Health
University of California
Davis, California

Reprint requests to:
Cathy L. Saiki, MS
Division of Occupational/
Environmental Medicine and
Epidemiology
Institute of Toxicology and
Environmental Health
University of California
Davis, CA 95616-8648

Development of company policies regarding workplace hazards to reproductive health requires an interdisciplinary approach, ideally with input from epidemiologists, toxicologists, occupational health physicians, industrial hygiene specialists, engineers, and human resources personnel. It is in the implementation of company policies in the workplace that many conflicts and complications may arise. Rights to be free of discrimination in the workplace may conflict with the right to be free of hazards to reproduction in the workplace for a given individual. Scientific knowledge of the risks to human reproduction of chemical, biological, and physical agents are often unknown or poorly understood. If data exist on risks to reproduction of any given agent, such data may be available for only one gender. Thus, such policies may of necessity be developed with incomplete and imperfect information. These policies are also influenced by economic demands and legal issues, making the development and implementation of such policies a complex task.

Paul et al.[17] made one of the few standardized attempts to describe workplace policies on reproductive hazards in the workplace. In a survey of 198 chemical and electronics manufacturing companies in Massachusetts, company representatives were asked for information on the following 3 areas: (1) company awareness of any reproductive hazards in the workplace; (2) health and safety education available to workers; and (3) existence of policies for job transfer or

TABLE 1. Elements of a Workplace Policy on Hazards to Reproductive Health

Hazard Definition	Employee Notification and Training
Exposure Assessment	Counseling of Affected Employees
Hazard Abatement	Employment Options for Affected Employees
Administrative Controls	Worksite Modifications
Engineering Controls	Voluntary Transfer or Reassignment
Work Practice Controls	Retention of Benefits and Seniority
Personal Protective Equipment	

exclusion of workers related to reproductive risks. Chemical companies were more likely than electronics companies to acknowledge the presence of substances associated with reproductive risk (46% vs. 38%). Larger firms were more aware of potential reproductive risks than were smaller firms. Being unionized was not related to awareness of potential reproductive hazards by the companies. Most companies (85%) reported some form of health and safety training for employees, most commonly right-to-know training or provision of material safety data sheets. Slightly fewer than half (89 of 198 firms) provided specific education related to *reproductive* risks; reproductive risk education was more common in larger firms.

In this chapter, we discuss the elements of a workplace policy and the legal and ethical issues related to workplace policy on reproductive hazards.

ELEMENTS OF WORKPLACE POLICY ON REPRODUCTIVE HAZARDS

Elements of workplace policy on reproductive hazards are summarized in Table 1.

Hazard Definition and Exposure Assessment

Employers first must become informed on the potential reproductive effects of agents used in their facilities and then develop strategies to address those hazards. In areas of known or suspect reproductive hazards, the presence and levels of exposures to employees first must be assessed.

Improvements in Industrial Hygiene Controls

The ideal solution to the presence of a reproductive risk in the workplace is elimination of exposure by complete removal of its source. This is best achieved by materials substitution, but care must be taken to avoid introducing materials with unknown reproductive toxicities. When removal or substitution is not feasible, a basic tenet of good industrial hygiene practice is to control the hazard as close to the source as possible.[26] Administrative controls, such as restricting time spent by employees in work areas with hazards to reproduction, also may be implemented to reduce exposures. The subsequent hierarchy of optimum controls is: first, engineering controls; second, work practice controls; and finally, personal protective equipment.

Companies can implement toxics use reduction programs for reproductive hazards in order to reduce the use of toxic chemicals and the generation of toxic wastes.[6] The industrial hygiene staff would inventory and analyze the use of chemicals or biologic agents hazardous to reproduction and would seek ways to reduce or eliminate the use of these agents. Technical options could include process or design changes, chemical substitutions, product redesign, improvements in operations and maintenance, and within-process recycling and reuse. As of

1991, 12 states had passed toxics use reduction or pollution prevention laws; agents hazardous to reproduction should be targeted as these laws are implemented in the workplace and in the overall environment.

Communication to Employees of Information on Reproductive Hazards

Employees have a legal and ethical right to know about hazards they face in the workplace.[2,14] Employers are required in several sections of the Occupational Safety and Health Act[16] to (1) use labels or warnings as necessary to apprise employees of risks to which they are exposed (sec. 5); (2) notify employees who have been or are exposed to toxic materials or harmful physical agents at levels exceeding occupational safety and health standards [sec. 8 (c)(3)]; and (3) inform employees of imminent dangers [sec. 13 (c)].

Informing employees of reproductive hazards in the workplace is complicated by, in many cases, a lack of valid scientific information on the impact of many agents on reproduction in one or both sexes.[13] In the absence of such information, employees should be told of the uncertainties and that having no evidence of harm is not the same as knowing that a substance is safe. If guidelines are based on extrapolating the results of animal reproductive toxicology studies, that uncertainty should be revealed.

Employers may present information on reproductive hazards in the workplace at special or routine informational meetings, safety training sessions, or other occasions. Employees should be instructed as to how compliance with safety procedures and use of personal protective equipment can reduce their exposures.

Counseling of Potentially Affected Employees

Resources for counseling employees about reproductive health hazards vary considerably among companies.[11] Larger companies may have occcupational health professionals, epidemiologists, industrial hygienists, and toxicologists available to employees, while small workplaces may have a limited ability to provide assistance. Counseling needs may be especially acute following workplace notifications of potential risks. It is important that a support network be in place to provide additional information, answer individual concerns, discuss worksite evaluations, and provide information about job transfer policies.

The employee may seek advice from his or her personal health care provider about workplace reproductive hazards, but most providers lack the training or awareness of the issues involved to provide good counseling.[20] Companies can provide employees with materials to give their providers to help them become more sensitive to the risks encountered by their patients in the workplace. Providers approached by at-risk employees need access to information on exposures, occupational medical consultation, and up-to-date toxicologic and epidemiologic information that would allow them to counsel patients effectively. However, providers such as primary care physicians face stringent time contraints that may prevent them from providing a quality response to patient requests.[20] Physicians can translate into lay terms information about the risks and place those risks in perspective to nonoccupational risks such as advanced maternal age, smoking, and previous history of pregnancy loss.[7] When supplied with appropriate knowledge, concerned physicians can play a pivotal role in helping workers reach informed decisions regarding employment and reproductive risks.

Job Transfers, Reassignments, Job Security

Job transfers or reassignments are made at the discretion of the employer, or they may be voluntary—at the request of the employee because of his or her concern about reproductive hazards in the workplace. Employers often require employees requesting voluntary transfers to provide a physician's request for the transfer. Issues of concern to employees and employers include wage retention after a transfer, reinstatement to the former position if the relocation is temporary, maintenance of seniority or promotion pathways, and the skill level of the job reassigned to the employee. The availability of paid or unpaid leaves of absence relating to avoidance of reproductive risks during critical times should be addressed, as well as whether employees retain benefits during leave periods.

In Finland, a maternity leave act became effective in 1991 that allows women who are exposed to agents considered harmful to pregnancy or the offspring to request a transfer to another job from the beginning of pregnancy.[24] If a job without exposures is not available, the woman may be eligible for a special maternity leave and benefits. The occupational physician is responsible for assessing whether the exposure is a hazard to the pregnancy or the offspring according to a list of agents accompanying the legislation. The level of exposure, not just the presence or absence of the agent in the workplace, is considered, and the guidelines accompanying the legislation also suggest the level of the exposure considered harmful.

Screening, Monitoring, Surveillance, and Medical Removal Protection

Medical screening in the workplace can be used to select and maintain a work force based on medical criteria.[22] Screening can be used to predict future risk of disease (predictive screening) or to assess current fitness for employment based on factors such as genetics, gender, age, lifestyle practices, general health status, or previous occupational exposure.

If hazards to reproduction are known, companies might implement surveillance programs to monitor exposure levels in the work environment and personal exposure levels of employees. This monitoring can alert employers and employees to exposures greater than action levels (levels lower than standards but requiring further monitoring) or permissible exposure levels. Further monitoring or risk reduction procedures may be required. However, levels frequently are developed without consideration of risks to reproduction. Such levels may not ensure the safety of persons trying to conceive, pregnant women, and their offspring.

Biologic monitoring can be undertaken to assess the exposure and uptake of toxic substances by workers and the biologic effects on those workers. Companies might be required to conduct periodic medical surveillance such as periodic medical examinations or laboratory testing to detect adverse health effects in workers known to be exposed to certain hazards. Under health standards promulgated under OSHA,[16] medical removal protection may be instituted if an employee's monitoring results reach some defined threshold. Medical removal protection for reproductive health hazards is of doubtful value because threshold levels may be too high to protect reproduction, and lag times between monitoring, and removal likely will occur too late to prevent reproductive damage. Medical removal triggered by knowledge of a pregnancy may fail to protect the fetus during the vulnerable first 6–8 weeks of development, when exposure to a reproductive toxicant can result in a spontaneous abortion or congenital malformation. Also, some firms require that a physician request removal during pregnancy, which further may delay removal. Policies of medical removal of pregnant women from hazardous sites provide no protection to the offspring from reproductive toxicants affecting men.

LEGAL AND ETHICAL ISSUES RELATED TO WORKPLACE POLICIES ON REPRODUCTIVE HEALTH

The development and implementation of employer policies on the protection of reproductive health involve complex issues of both science and law. Worthwhile and important goals such as safety from reproductive hazards and freedom from discrimination on the basis of gender or pregnancy may often conflict. The issues of reproductive hazards in the workplace may cause the intrusion of employers into the very personal area of employees' reproductive status and plans. The employee's privacy may be invaded, and information that might otherwise be confidential may of necessity be known in the workplace.

Legal Causation

Proving causation in courts of law requires that the plaintiff show with a preponderance of evidence that the exposure more likely than not caused the adverse health outcome.[15] Judges and juries in these cases often are presented with complex and unfamiliar technical information. The Henle-Koch Postulates may be of use in proving causation in tort cases of liability. However, because the postulates were largely designed for assessing causation in large groups, the criteria must be adapted to determine the probability of causation in individual cases. Definitive proof of causation likely will be impossible; therefore, determining what legal criteria are acceptable to prove harm is a complex task. Epidemiologic evidence may suggest trends in disease occurrence related to exposures in populations, but interpreting and extrapolating population trends and probabilities to the level of the individual is difficult.

Identification of a Population at Increased Risk

Medical surveillance and exposure monitoring of employees in the workplace may identify groups of workers who are at greater risk or more susceptible to harm from workplace hazards.[1,5] Without regulatory restraints, often the motivation behind medical screening and surveillance is to exclude from the workplace individuals most likely to experience occupational injury and disease. Such employees may cause increased costs to employers through medical and legal claims.[19,22] Such screening also may prove discriminatory if certain classes (e.g., gender) of workers are affected differently. Reducing exposures in the workplace is an alternative that initially may be more costly to employers but ultimately may result in reduced medical and legal costs as well as a healthier and more productive work force.

Informing workers of their health risks from exposure to toxic substances in the workplace may yield claims of employment discrimination, psychological harm or stress,[10] economic impacts, and other effects. Stigmatization of the "at-risk" worker also may occur.[23]

Gender Discrimination

Title VII of the 1964 Civil Rights Act[25] in part states that "it shall be an unlawful employment practice for an employer . . . to limit, segregate, or classify his employees . . . in any way which would deprive or tend to deprive any individual of employment opportunities or otherwise adversely affect his status as an employee, because of such individual's race, color, religion, sex, or national origin." Discriminating against a woman because of her pregnancy or fertility status was not upheld by the courts to be covered by Title VII; therefore, in 1978, an amendment to Title VII, known as the Pregnancy Discrimination Act, was added. The amendment expanded the definition of "on the basis of sex" to include . . . "because of or on the basis of pregnancy, childbirth, or related medical conditions." Thus, a woman cannot be denied employment or removed from employment because of her reproductive health status.

Exclusionary and Fetal Protection Policies

In the survey of companies conducted in 1987 by Paul and colleagues,[17] about one fifth of 198 firms responded affirmatively to the query of whether they ever "restrict(s) any workers from working with certain substances or in areas or occupations which may affect reproductive health." Of 58 total restrictions by 37 companies, most (67%) were applied to pregnant women, while only 1 of 58 restrictions was applied to male workers (whose partners were trying to conceive). Of the 28 companies that restricted pregnant women, most offered job transfer or a leave of absence.

In 1991, the U.S. Supreme Court unanimously ruled that the exclusion of women of childbearing age from jobs with risks to reproduction via actual or potential lead exposure in a battery manufacturing plant exceeding the OSHA standard was facially discriminatory under Title VII of the Civil Rights Act of 1964 as amended in the 1978 Pregnancy Discrimination Act.[12,18] This action came in response to a policy initiated in 1982 by Johnson Controls. After eight of its employees became pregnant while having blood lead levels exceeding the OSHA standard, Johnson Controls instituted a policy barring all women, except those whose infertility was medically documented, from jobs having actual or potential lead exposure exceeding the OSHA standard. The policy did not apply to male workers, despite evidence about the debilitating effects of lead on the male reproductive system. A group including affected employees filed a class action petition in the District Court claiming that the policy constituted sex discrimination. The District Court and, subsequently, the Court of Appeals granted judgment for the respondent, Johnson Controls, on the basis that the policy constituted a business necessity and was reasonably necessary to further the industrial safety concern that was part of the essence of its business. This exclusionary policy, which is now commonly known as a fetal protection policy, was shown to discriminate explicitly against women on the basis of their sex[4,8,9] and resulted in the U.S. Supreme Court in 1991 overturning these lower court rulings.

Voluntary Assumption of Risk

At times employees may be given the opportunity or encouraged to assume the responsibility for risk of exposure to reproductive hazards in the workplace. Employees may feel compelled to continue working after they have been informed that the work environment harbors reproductive hazards. Subtle psychologic pressures from superiors and/or pressing economic need may cause employees to expose themselves to risks they would not otherwise undertake. Does an informed employee assume responsibility for detriment caused by known reproductive hazards in the workplace? Does an informed employee have cause for recourse with the employer if reproductive injury should occur?

In the wake of the Supreme Court's ruling on the Johnson Controls case,[12] some employers did not absolutely exclude fertile women from jobs with reproductive hazards, but instead used means to discourage women (but not men) from working in such jobs.[3] Some companies that had fetal protection policies have not made any process or engineering changes that would lessen or remove the reproductive hazard. Instead, they have sought waivers from any fertile women who work in jobs previously covered by an exclusionary policy.

Under the Occupational Safety and Health Act,[16] the employer has a duty to provide a place of employment free from recognized hazards likely to cause serious physical harm to employees. Any company that previously had a fetal protection policy (a recognized hazard) and then sought to transfer the responsibility for the risk to the employee without taking affirmative steps to remove or mitigate the risk would appear to violate the Occupational Safety and Health Act.[3]

Workers' Compensation

State workers' compensation statutes cover most private sector workers,[19] but recovery under workers' compensation statutes for reproductive harm is generally not successful. An adult worker often has only the avenue of workers' compensation for recovery for occupational injury and disease, but reproductive harm is generally not covered by workers' compensation statutes.[3] State laws vary, but there are three major requirements that affect a worker's ability to secure recompense for reproductive harm: (1) "personal" injury or disease; (2) the injury or disease must result in job disability; and (3) the injury or disease must be caused by a workplace accident or exposure.[26] In most states, the "personal" criterion for injury or disease prevents claims for harms to the developing fetus. Unless the worker experiences specified types of disability, he or she often will not qualify for benefits based on lost or diminished sexual or reproductive functions. Also the injury or disease must be shown to be job-related. Reproductive problems such as infertility that also may occur from nonoccupational causes may not be accepted as having been caused by an exposure at work.

A worker's spouse, children, or future children are not covered by workers' compensation protection. Therefore, in cases of reproductive injury or disease or damage to offspring, the judicial tort system may be the only avenue for recourse. Often, state workers' compensation statutes forbid recovery through the judicial system, known as the exclusivity of remedy doctrine, but in some states this doctrine has been relaxed in limited circumstances.[26] Tort actions are generally an available avenue if workers' compensation laws do not apply to the situation.

Trends in Litigation Outcomes

In toxic torts cases, providing a preponderance of evidence for causation of reproductive harm has proved difficult.[15] Trends toward easing the requirements for proof, especially in cases of population exposures, have resulted in a portion of the burden of proof on the plaintiffs being shifted to the defendant or in the allowance of claims for risk of future injury or emotional distress. Even when the best objective epidemiologic and medical evidence is presented, often the credibility and presentation of expert witnesses is more convincing to a lay jury than scientific validity and quality.

Clauss et al., state that the legal system "... has a tendency to deal with societal problems in an incremental, subdivided way that can be frustrating to those seeking an immediate, global answer. To work within that system, litigants are constrained to proceed in a measured fashion in structuring their lawsuits and often cannot rely on litigation alone to reach the ultimate goal."[3] The issue decided in International Union UAW versus Johnson Controls, Inc. was a first step in the direction of securing freedom from discrimination in issues of reproductive safety in the workplace. Now the task must be to pursue the goal of a safe workplace for women and men in terms of their reproductive health.[21]

SUMMARY

At present, workplace policies regarding reproductive hazards are not regulated directly, and inappropriate policies are occasionally corrected by legal actions or union pressures on the employers. Further, information on reproductive hazards is incomplete; however, employees have a legal right to know available information about hazards, including reproductive hazards, that they face in the workplace. Occupational health personnel play a major role in communicating information about reproductive hazards in the workplace and in implementing company policy and complying with legislation. Regulatory and case law likely will continue to evolve as many issues related to safety from reproductive hazards in the workplace have not yet been resolved.

REFERENCES

1. Atherley G, Johnston N, Tennassee M: Biomedical surveillance: Rights conflict with rights. J Occup Med 28:958–965, 1986.
2. Bayer R: Notifying workers at risk: The politics of the right-to-know. Am J Publ Health 76:1352–1356, 1986.
3. Clauss CA, Berzon M, Bertin J: Litigating reproductive and developmental health in the aftermath of UAW versus Johnson Controls. Environ Health Perspect 101(suppl 2):205–220, 1993.
4. Daniels C, Paul M, Rosofsky R: Health, equity, and reproductive risks in the workplace. J Public Health Policy 11:449–462, 1990.
5. Draper E: Risky business. Genetic Testing and Exclusionary Practices in the Hazardous Workplace. New York, Cambridge University Press, 1991.
6. Geiser K: Protecting reproductive health and the environment: Toxics use reduction. Environ Health Perspect 101(suppl 2):221–225, 1993.
7. Giacoia GP: Reproductive hazards in the workplace. Obstet Gynecol Surv 47:679–687, 1992.
8. Graham T, Lessin N, Mirer F: A labor perspective on workplace reproductive hazards: Past history, current concerns, and positive directions. Environ Health Perspect 101(suppl 2):199–204, 1993.
9. Hoadley DL: Fetal protection policies. Effective tools for gender discrimination. J Legal Med 12:85–104, 1991.
10. Houts PS, McDougall V: Effects of informing workers of their health risks from exposure to toxic materials. Am J Ind Med 13:271–279, 1988.
11. Hunt PE: Reproductive health issues. Workplace perspectives. Am Assoc Occup Health Nurs J 40:72–77, 1992.
12. International Union, United Automobile, Aerospace and Agricultural Implement Workers of America, et al. v. Johnson Controls, Inc., 111 S. Ct. 1196–1217, 1991.
13. Johnston JD, Jamieson GG, Wright S: Reproductive and developmental hazards and employment policies. Br J Ind Med 49:85–94, 1992.
14. Millar JD: The right to know in the workplace. The moral dimension. Ann N Y Acad Sci 572:113–121, 1989.
15. Muscat JE, Huncharek MS: Causation and disease: Biomedical science in toxic tort litigation. J Occup Med 31:997–1002, 1989.
16. Occupational Safety and Health Act. 29 USC, sec. 651 et seq.
17. Paul M, Daniels C, Rosofsky R: Corporate response to reproductive hazards in the workplace: Results of the family, work, and health survey. Am J Ind Med 16:267–280, 1989.
18. Pregnancy Discrimination Act of 1978. 42 USC, sec. 2000e et seq.
19. Raines LJ: Biological testing and occupational disease liability. J Occup Med 28:921–923, 1986.

20. Rest KM: Is the medical community ready for worker notification? Am J Ind Med 23:25–32, 1993.
21. Robinson JC, Giacomini MK: A reallocation of rights in industries with reproductive health hazards. The Milbank Quarterly 70:587–603, 1992.
22. Rothstein MA: Discriminatory aspects of medical screening. J Occup Med 28:924–929, 1986.
23. Sands RG, Newby LG, Greenberg RA: Labeling of health risk in industrial settings. J Appl Behav Sci 17:359–374, 1981.
24. Taskinen H: Prevention of reproductive health hazards at work. Scand J Work Environ Health 18(suppl 2):27–29, 1992.
25. Title VII of the Civil Rights Act, Public Law 88–352, July 2, 1964. 42 USC, sec. 2000e-2(a)(1).
26. U.S. Congress, Office of Technology Assessment: Reproductive hazards in the workplace. Washington, DC: US Govt Printing Office, 1986, publication OTA-BA-266.

INDEX

Entries in **boldface** type indicate complete articles.

Abortion, spontaneous, occupational exposure-
  related, 424, 459–460, 472
  anesthetic gases exposure-related, 368, 456,
    457
  antineoplastic drug exposure-related, 457,
    460
  electrical industry employment-related, 447,
    453, 460
  electromagnetic field exposure-related,
    442–446, 459
  glycol ether exposure-related, 459–460
  health care employment-related, 368, 454,
    455, 456–457, 460
  hydrocarbon exposure-related, 449, 459–460
  lead exposure-related, 367, 454, 460
  literature review of, 442–458
  mercury exposure-related, 454, 455
  metals exposure-related, 514, 522–525
  methodologic issues related to, 439, 459
  population-based studies of, 406, 407
  prevalence of, 365
  recurrent, 420–421
  of unknown etiology, 364
  urinary assays for detection of, 425–426
Adenoma, prolactin-secreting, 417–418
Adenosine triphosphate, as sperm fertility
  marker, 398
Agricultural employment
  maternal, 368, 475, 482
    as preterm birth risk factor, 462
    as spontaneous abortion risk factor,
      460
    paternal, as congenital abnormalities risk
      factor, 486
Air Contaminant Standards (Occupational
  Safety and Health Administration),
  378–379
Alcohol use, spermatogenesis-impairing effect
  of, 389
American Conference of Governmental
  Industrial Hygienists, 374, 378, 379
Anesthetic gases
  maternal exposure to
    as congenital abnormalities risk factor,
      476, 478
    as spontaneous abortion risk factor, 368,
      456, 457
    as subfertility risk factor, 368
  paternal exposure to, as congenital
    abnormalities risk factor, 476
Animal screening tests, 375–376
Antibiotics, as infertility risk factor, 439, 441

Antineoplastic drugs, maternal exposure to
  as congenital abnormalities risk factor, 475,
    476
  as spontaneous abortion risk factor, 457, 460
Antisperm antibody tests, 398–399
Arsenic
  as menstrual disorder risk factor, 438
  paternal exposure to, 367
Artificial insemination, 366
Asherman's syndrome, 416–417

Benzene, paternal exposure to, 481, 490
Biologic monitoring, of workplace reproductive
  hazards, 544
Birth Defects Prevention Act, 381
Bladder surgery, as retrograde ejaculation
  cause, 389
Brain tumors, in children, parental
  occupational exposure-related, 495
  agricultural employment-related, 514,
    518–519
  manufacturing chemicals exposure-related,
    499, 506–511, 514
  metals exposure-related, 514
  textiles exposure-related, 515, 527–528
  wood-related occupations employment-
    related, 531–532
n-Butyl acetate, as menstrual disorder risk
  factor, 438

Cadmium
  maternal exposure to, 464–465
  paternal exposure to, 367
Cancer therapy, as infertility risk factor, 389
Carbaryl, paternal exposure to, 367
Cardiovascular abnormalities
  maternal occupational exposure-related,
    478, 481
  paternal occupational exposure-related,
    490–491
Case-control studies
  of childhood cancer, 496, 498–499
  of congenital abnormalities, 472
  of female infertility, 437
  limitations of, 491
  of maternal occupational exposure, 476–484
  of paternal occupational exposure, 407–408,
    487–491
  recall bias in, 408
  of spontaneous abortion, 439, 442–443, 444,
    445, 448–449, 450, 453, 457

551

Central nervous system tumors. *See* Nervous
    system tumors
Ceramics industry employment, as low
    birthweight risk factor, 464
Chemicals. *See also* specific chemicals
    maternal exposure to, 483
    paternal exposure to, 367
Chernobyl nuclear radiation disaster, 405–406.
    See also Radiation
Childbearing age, extension of, 366
Childhood cancer, parental occupational
    exposure-related, **495–539**
    electromagnetic field exposure-related
        cancers, 535–536
    farming and agricultural exposure-related
        cancers, 514, 516–520
    hydrocarbon exposure-related cancers, 489,
        499–514
    metals exposure-related cancers, 514,
        522–525
    methodologic issues in, 496–499
    petroleum exposure-related cancers, 499–514
    population-based studies of, 406
    radiation exposure-related cancers, 515, 521,
        529, 534–535
    solvents exposure-related cancers, 499–514
    textiles exposure-related cancers, 514,
        526–528
    wood, paper and pulp exposure-related
        cancers, 514, 532–533
Cimetidine, spermatogenesis-impairing effect
    of, 389
Civil Rights Act of 1964
    fetal protection policies and, 380
    Title VII, 545–546
        Pregnancy Discrimination Act
            amendment of, 368–369, 380, 546
Clinical (case) studies, of paternal occupational
    exposure, 410–411
Cocaine, spermatogenesis-impairing effect of,
    389
Cohort studies
    of female infertility, 437
    limitations of, 410, 491
    of paternal occupational exposure, 408–410,
        485–486
    pregnancy, 472
        of maternal occupational exposure,
            474–475
        of paternal occupational exposure,
            485–486
    of spontaneous abortion, 439, 443, 444, 445,
        446, 449, 450, 451, 452, 454, 455–456,
        457, 458
Cold temperatures, as menstrual disorder risk
    factor, 438
Conception, monthly possibility of, 388, 415
Congenital adrenal hyperplasia, 417
Congenital malformations, parental
    occupational exposure-related, **471–494**
    antenatal diagnosis of, 421, 422

Congenital malformations, parental
    occupational exposure-related *(cont.)*
    exposure assessment and groupings of,
        472–473
    linked registry data of, 474
    maternal exposure studies of, 474–484
        case-control studies, 476–484
        occupational cohort studies, 475–476
        pregnancy cohort studies, 474–475
        registry-based studies, 474
    mutation-related, 365
    outcome classification and groupings of,
        473–474
    paternal exposure studies of, 472, 474,
        484–492
        case-control studies, 477–478,
            487–491
        occupational cohort studies, 476,
            486–487
        population-based studies, 406
        pregnancy cohort studies, 485–486
        registry-based studies, 484–485
    prevalence of, 365
    of unknown etiology, 364
Counseling programs, for workplace
    reproductive hazards, 543
Creatine phosphokinase, as sperm maturity
    marker, 398
Cross-sectional studies
    of paternal exposure, 408, 410
    of spontaneous abortion, 439, 446, 447–448,
        451, 452, 454
Cryptorchidism, as infertility risk factor, 389
Cushing's syndrome, 417

DDT, as gonadotropin inhibitor, 365
Death certificates, use in childhood cancer
    studies, 497–498
Dehydroepiandrosterone sulfate, as androgen-
    secreting tumor marker, 417
Developmental toxicants, federal government's
    list of, 379, 380
Developmental toxicity
    animal screening study guidelines for,
        375–376
    differentiated from reproductive toxicity,
        378
    endpoints in, 471–472
    male-mediated, 472
Dexamethasone suppression test, 417
Diabetes mellitus, as infertility risk factor,
    389
Dibromochloropropane
    paternal exposure to, as infertility cause,
        367, 405
    Permissible Exposure Levels for, 374, 378
    as spermatotoxin, 365
Dinitrotoluene, 406
Dinosep, ban of, 375
Dioxin, as low birthweight risk factor, 464

Discrimination. *See also* Pregnancy
  Discrimination Act
  gender-related, 545–546
  toxic exposure-related, 545
Dose-response effects, mathematical modeling
  of, 378
Dose-response fallacy, 483
Down syndrome, paternal occupational
  exposure-related, 484–485, 490
Drinking water
  California state regulations for, 369,
    382–384
  organic solvents-contaminated, 464
Dry cleaning workers
  infertility in, 439, 440
  spontaneous abortion in, 449
Dyes, maternal exposure to, 479
  as infertility risk factor, 439, 440

Early fetal loss (EFL). *See also* Abortion,
    spontaneous
  undetected, 366
  urinary assays for detection of, 425–426
Electrical industry employment. *See also*
    Electromagnetic fields
  as low birthweight risk factor, 464
  as preterm birth risk factor, 462
  as spontaneous abortion risk factor, 447,
    453, 460
Electric blankets
  as low birthweight risk factor, 463–464
  as spontaneous abortion risk factor, 446
Electromagnetic fields
  maternal exposure to
    as low birthweight risk factor, 463
    as spontaneous abortion risk factor,
      442–446, 459
  paternal exposure to, as childhood cancer
    risk factor, 515, 535–536
Embryo transfer, 366
Endometriosis, as infertility risk factor, 416,
    418, 419–420
Endpoints, reproductive
  in risk assessment, 376–378
  for women, 368
Environmental Protection Agency (EPA), 374
  risk assessment guidelines of, 376, 377
Epididymis, physical examination of, 390
Estradiol, metabolism of, 427
Estradiol glucuronide, as ovulation biomarker,
    430
Estradiol metabolites, urinary assays of, 427,
    430–431
Estrogen, relationship to infertility, 416–418
Estrogen agonists/antagonists, 365
Estrogen metabolites, urinary assays of,
    429–431
Estrone glucuronide, as ovulation biomarker,
    430
Ethoxyacetic acid, paternal exposure to, 367

Ethoxyethanol, Permissible Exposure Levels
    for, 379
Ethoxyethanol acetate
  paternal exposure to, 367
  Permissible Exposure Levels for, 379
Ethylene dibromide, paternal exposure to, 367
Ethylene glycol, as spontaneous abortion cause,
    446
Ethylene glycol ethers. *See also* Glycol ethers
  reproductive toxicity of, 367
Ethylene oxide, 373
  Permissible Exposure Levels for, 374

Fecundability, 415
Fecundability ratio, 435
Federal Insecticide, Fungicide, and Rodenticide
    Act (FIFRA), 374–375, 381
Fertility, indicators for, 435, 436
Fertility ratio, standardized, 436
  birth rate overestimation by, 408
Fetal alcohol syndrome, 422
Fetal protection policies
  as job discrimination, 546
  lawsuits related to, 379–381
  risk assumption in, 547
Fibroids, uterine, as infertility risk factor, 420
Flight attendants
  premature births to, 462
  spontaneous abortion in, 444, 459
Fluoride, as menstrual disorder risk factor, 437
Follicle-stimulating hormone
  in male infertility, 399
  in menstrual dysfunction, 417–418
  urinary assays for, 431
Food processing industry employment, paternal
  occupational exposure in, 486

Gamete intrafallopian transfer (GIFT), 420
General Accounting Office (GAO),
    reproductive toxicants report of,
    365–366, 379, 380
Genetic disorders, antenatal diagnosis of, 421–422
Germ cell tumors, parental occupational
    exposure-related, 513
Germicides, maternal exposure to, as
    spontaneous abortion risk factor, 460
Glycol ethers, 373
  as menstrual disorder risk factor, 438
  Permissible Exposure Levels for, 375,
    378–379
  as spontaneous abortion risk factor, 459–460

Hairdressers, menstrual disorders in, 438
Health care employment
  as congenital abnormalities risk factor,
    477–478
  as spontaneous abortion risk factor, 368,
    454, 455, 456–457, 460
  as subfertility risk factor, 368

Heat, paternal exposure to, 367, 368
Heavy metals, paternal exposure to, 367, 368
Henle-Koch Postulates, 545
Hepatoblastoma, parental occupational
    exposure-related, 513, 514, 525
Herbicide exposure, effect on semen quality,
    367
Hiroshima survivors, children of, 521, 529
HLA typing, for infertility evaluation, 421
Human chorionic gonadotropin (hCG), as early
    fetal loss indicator, 425–426, 429–430
Hydrocarbons
    maternal exposure to, as spontaneous
        abortion risk factor, 449, 459–460
    parental exposure to, as childhood cancer
        risk factor, 499–514
    paternal exposure to, 367
        as congenital abnormalities risk factor,
            485, 488–489, 491–492
Hyperandrogenism, as female infertility risk
    factor, 417
Hypertension, pregnancy-induced, 465
Hypogonadism, hypogonadotropic, 399
Hypoosmotic swelling test, 396

Immunobead test, 398–399
Industrial hygiene controls, 542–543
Infant mortality rate, 365
Infertility, 439, 440–441
    definition of, 415
    duration of, 388
    female, clinical approach to, **415–422**
        cervical factors evaluation, 420
        coordination with partners' clinical
            evaluation, 388
        immunologic factors evaluation, 420
        ovulatory dysfunction evaluation,
            415–418
        tubal/pelvic factors evaluation, 418–420
        uterine factors evaluation, 420
    increase of, 365
    male, clinical approach to, **387–404**
        clinical diagnostic tests, 399
        clinical evaluation, 388–390
        endocrine evaluation, 399
        semen evaluation, 388, 390–399
    prevalence of, 438–439
    treatment cost for, 364
    unexplained, 415, 420
International Union of United Auto Workers v.
    Johnson Controls, 379, 381, 546, 547, 548
Intrauterine growth retardation, 462–463, 464
In vitro fertilization, 366
    sperm function bioassay for, 397, 398
In vitro fertilization and embryo transfer
    (IVF-ET), 419, 420–421

Job exposure matrix (JEM), 473
Job titles, as occupational exposure
    classification method, 407, 473

Job transfer/reassignment, for reproductive
    hazard avoidance, 544, 546
Johnson Controls, Inc., fetal protection policy-
    related lawsuit against, 379, 381, 546,
    547, 548

Kepone
    as estrogen agonist/antagonist, 365
    paternal exposure to, 411

Lacquers, maternal/conceptus exposure to, 479
Lead, occupational exposure to, 373
    maternal exposure, 480
        fetal protection policies for, 380, 546
        as low birthweight risk factor, 464–465
        as pregnancy-induced hypertension risk
            factor, 465
        as preterm birth risk factor, 462
        as spontaneous abortion risk factor, 454,
            460
    OSHA standard for, 380
    paternal exposure, 487, 490–491
        as congenital abnormalities risk factor,
            367
        historical background of, 405
        as infertility risk factor, 410–411
        as spontaneous abortion risk factor,
            367
    Permissible Exposure Levels for, 374
United Auto Workers v. *Johnson Controls,
    Inc.*, 379, 381, 546, 547, 548
Leather-working industry employment, as low
    birthweight risk factor, 464
Leukemia, parental occupational exposure-
    related
    acute lymphocytic, 495
    agricultural employment-related, 514,
        516–518
    manufacturing chemicals exposure-related,
        499, 501–506
    metals exposure-related, 522–524
    radiation exposure-related, 488, 521, 529,
        534–535
    textiles exposure-related, 515, 526–527
    wood-related occupations employment-
        related, 530–531
Liver disease, as infertility risk factor, 389
Longitudinal studies, 410
Low birthweight, occupational exposure-
    related, 462–465
Low birthweight infants, annual number of,
    364
Lubricating oils, as infertility risk factor, 439,
    440
Luteal phase defect, 421
Luteinizing hormone
    as early fetal loss indicator, 425–426,
        429–430
    in male infertility, 399
    urinary assays for, 431

Lymphoma, parental occupational exposure-related
  agricultural employment-related, 514, 516–518
  manufacturing chemicals exposure-related, 499, 501–506
  metals exposure-related, 522–524
  occupational exposure-related, 495
  radiation exposure-related, 521, 529, 534, 535
  textiles exposure-related, 515, 526–527
  wood-related occupations employment-related, 530–531

Male reproduction, occupational hazards to. *See* Paternal occupational exposure
Manufacturing industry employment, as low birthweight risk factor, 464
Marijuana, spermatogenesis-impairing effect of, 389
Maternity leave, 544
Medical removal protection, for reproductive health hazards, 544–545
Medical screening programs, 544, 545
Menstrual cycle
  as ovulatory function measure, 427–428, 436–437
  progesterone measurement during, 428–429
Menstrual dysfunction, occupational exposure-related, 437–438
  follicle-stimulating hormone levels in, 417–418
Mercury
  maternal exposure to
    as low birthweight risk factor, 464
    as spontaneous abortion risk factor, 454, 455
    as menstrual disorder risk factor, 438, 460
  paternal exposure to, 367, 489
Metals
  maternal exposure to
    as infertility risk factor, 439, 440, 454–455, 460
    as low birthweight risk factor, 464
    as preterm birth risk factor, 462
  parental exposure to, as childhood cancer risk factor, 514, 522–525
Methoxyethanol
  paternal exposure to, 367
  Permissible Exposure Levels for, 379
Methoxyethanol acetate
  paternal exposure to, 367
  Permissible Exposure Levels for, 379
Microwave diathermy, as spontaneous abortion risk factor, 442, 459
Multigenerational studies, 376, 378
Mumps, as orchitis cause, 389

Nagasaki survivors, children of, 521, 529
National Institute for Occupational Safety and Health
  occupational exposure standard-setting role of, 374
  Recommended Exposure Levels of, 378
Nervous system tumors, parental occupational exposure-related
  agricultural employment-related, 514, 518–519
  electromagnetic fields exposure-related, 535–536
  manufacturing chemicals exposure-related, 499, 506–511, 514
  textiles exposure-related, 515, 527–528
  wood-related occupations employment-related, 531–532
Neural tube defects, parental occupational exposure-related, 478, 486, 487–488, 489, 490
  antenatal diagnosis of, 421
  prevention of, 422
Neuroblastoma, paternal electromagnetic exposure-related, 535, 536
Neuroendocrine studies, of male reproductive system, 410
Night work, maternal, as preterm birth risk factor, 461
Nitrofurandantoin, spermatogenesis-impairing effect of, 389
Nitrous oxide, maternal exposure to, 368
  as infertility risk factor, 439, 441, 455
Noise
  maternal exposure to
    as infertility risk factor, 439, 440
    as low birthweight risk factor, 463
    as pregnancy-induced hypertension risk factor, 465
    as menstrual disorder risk factor, 460
  paternal exposure to, 368
Nuclear industry, paternal radiation exposure in, 487–488, 521, 529, 534–535

Occupational cohort studies, 472
  of maternal exposure, 475–476
  of paternal exposure, 476, 486–487
Occupational exposure
  classified by job title, 407, 473, 499
  employees' voluntary risk assumption for, 546–547
  overlapping, 499
  prevalence of, 363
Occupational Safety and Health Act, 373–374
  risk assumption violations of, 547
Occupational Safety and Health Administration
  Lead Standard of, 380
  Permissible Exposure Levels of, 378–379
Oocyte, donor, 418

Organochlorines, as estrogen agonists/
   antagonists, 365
Ovarian function
   impairment/failure of, 418
      as infertility risk factor, 415–416, 424
      relationship to menstrual cycle, 427–428
Ovarian hormone metabolites, urinary assays
      of, 424, 426–431
   of estrogen metabolites, 429–431
   of progesterone metabolites, 428–429
Ovulation, urinary steroid assays of, 426–431
Oxydemoton-methyl, maternal exposure to, 482

Paints
   maternal exposure to, 479, 480
      as spontaneous abortion risk factor, 451
   parental exposure to, as childhood cancer
      risk factor, 499–514
   paternal exposure to, 485
Paternal occupational exposure, 367–368,
      405–414
   case-control studies of, 407–408, 477–478,
      487–491
   clinical studies of, 410–411
   cohort studies of, 408–410, 476, 486–487
   as congenital abnormalities risk factor, 366,
      472, 474, 484–492
      case-control studies of, 477–478, 487–491
      occupational cohort studies of, 476,
         486–487
      pregnancy-cohort studies of, 485–486
      registry-based studies of, 484–485
   implications for fetal protection policies, 381
   as infertility risk factor, 366
   to physical agents, as childhood cancer risk
      factor, 515, 521, 529, 534–537
   population-based studies of, 367, 406–407
   as spontaneous abortion risk factor, 450,
      451, 452, 456
   effect on semen quality, 367
   standardized fertility ratio for, 408
   surveillance programs for, 411
Pelvic inflammatory disease, as infertility risk
      factor, 418–419
Penis, physical examination of, 390
Perchloroethylene
   as menstrual disorder risk factor, 438
   as spontaneous abortion risk factor,
      459–460
Peritubal adhesions, as infertility risk factor,
      418–420
Permissible Exposure Levels (PELs)
   federal regulation of, 374
   for glycol ethers, 378–379
Personal protective equipment, 542
Pesticides
   California state regulations for, 381
   federal regulations for, 374–375
   maternal exposure to, 482–483
      as preterm birth risk factor, 462

Pesticides, maternal exposure to *(cont.)*   as
      spontaneous abortion risk factor,
         452–453, 460
   parental exposure to, 373
      as childhood cancer risk factor, 514
   paternal exposure to, 367, 486, 489
Pesticides, 373
Petroleum products, parental exposure to,
      405
   as childhood cancer risk factor, 499–514
Pharmaceutical industry, maternal
      occupational exposure in, 475
Physical work load, maternal
   as congenital abnormalities risk factor, 484
   as low birthweight risk factor, 463
   as pregnancy-induced hypertension risk
      factor, 465
   as preterm birth risk factor, 368
   as spontaneous abortion risk factor, 368,
      457–458, 460
Physiotherapy, maternal exposure during, 483
Pituitary function, urinary assays of, 424, 431
Polybrominated biphenyls, as estrogen
      agonists/antagonists, 365
Polychlorinated biphenyls, as estrogen
      agonists/antagonists, 365
Polycystic ovarian syndrome, 417
Population-based studies
   of paternal occupational exposure, 406–407
   urine assay use in, **423–433**
      to detect early fetal loss, 368, 425–426
      to monitor ovarian function, 368,
         426–431
      to monitor pituitary function, 431
Postcoital test, 420
Pott, Percivall, 405
Poverty, demographics of, 364–365
Prader-Willi syndrome, 485, 488–489,
      491–492
Pregnancy
   ectopic, following tubal surgery, 419
   first, employment during, 364
   job discrimination related to, 368–369, 380,
      545–546
   job reassignments during, 544
   outcome measures of, 435
Pregnancy cohort studies, 472
   of maternal exposure, 474–475
   of paternal exposure, 485–486
Pregnancy Discrimination Act, 368–369, 380,
      546
Pregnanediol-3-glucuronide, urinary assays of,
      427, 428–430
Pregnant women, medical removal protection
      policies for, 544–546
Preterm births
   annual number of, 364
   occupational exposure-related, 460–462
   population-based studies of, 406
Printing industry, paternal exposure in,
      486–487

Proestrogen challenge test, 416
Progesterone metabolites, urinary assays of, 427, 428–429
Proposition 65, 369, 382–384
Pulp and paper industry, parental employment in, as childhood cancer risk factor, 515, 532–533

Questionnaire studies, of paternal occupational exposure, 409, 410

Radiation
  maternal exposure to, 478, 483, 487, 488
  paternal exposure to, 478, 487–488
    as childhood cancer risk factor, 515, 521, 529, 534–535
Recommended Exposure Levels, 378
Registry-based studies, 472, 474, 484–485
Regulations, for workplace reproductive health protection, **373–386**
  California state regulations, 381–384
  federal laws, 373–375
    inadequacy of, 366
    non-reproductive-related standards of, 363, 364
  federal policies and regulatory programs, 375–381
    for animal testing, 375–376
    fetal protection policies, 379–381
    for reproductive endpoints, 376–378
    reproductive toxicant classification and, 368–369
Renal disease, as infertility risk factor, 389
Reproduction, hormonal regulation of, 365
Reproductive assessment by continuous breeding (RACB) protocol, 376
Reproductive biology, advances in knowledge of, 365–366
Reproductive endpoints
  in risk assessment, 376–378
  in women, 368
Reproductive system, toxicant sensitivity of, 363
Reproductive technology, advances in, 366
Reproductive toxicants. *See also* specific reproductive toxicants
  criteria for classification of, 369
  cumulative effects of, in women, 365
  federally identified list of, 379, 380
  federal regulation of, 365–366
Reproductive toxicity
  EPA guidelines for, 377
  male, implications for fetal protection policies, 381
Reproductive toxicology, male-mediated mechanisms of, 365
Retinoblastoma, paternal occupational exposure-related, 513
  agricultural employment-related, 520
  metals exposure-related, 514, 525

Rhabdomyosarcoma, parental manufacturing chemicals exposure-related, 512
Risk assessment
  differentiated from risk management, 376
  reproductive endpoints in, 376–378
Risk management, 376
Rubber industry employment, as low birthweight risk factor, 464

Safe Drinking Water and Toxic Enforcement Act, 369 382–384
Salfalazine, spermatogenesis-impairing effect of, 389
Sarcoma, parental occupational exposure-related
  Ewing's bone, agricultural employment-related, 514, 520
  soft-tissue
    manufacturing chemicals exposure-related, 512
    textiles exposure-related, 515, 528
    wood-related occupations employment-related, 515, 533
Scrotal cancer, in chimney sweeps, 405
Semen analysis, 388, 390–399
  of acrosomal integrity and function, 396
  antisperm antibody tests, 398–399
  automated, 366, 391, 392, 393
  bioassays of sperm function, 396–398
  biochemical tests, 398
  interpretation of semen parameters, 393–395
  methodologic limitations of, 410
  microscopic, 391–393
  plasma membrane integrity, 395–396
  round cell evaluation, 392, 393
  semen volume, 394
  specimen collection techniques for, 390–391
  sperm-cervical mucus interaction, 397
  sperm morphology, 392–393, 394, 395
  sperm motility, 391–392, 394
  sperm numbers, 394
  sperm penetration assay, 397
  sperm-zone pellucida interaction, 396, 397–398
Semiconductor workers, spontaneous abortion in, 460
Service industry employment, as low birthweight risk factor, 464
Sex-hormone binding protein, 427
Sexual intercourse, frequent, effect on male fertility, 389
Sheehan's syndrome, 418
Shift work, maternal
  as low birthweight risk factor, 463
  as menstrual disorder risk factor, 438
  as pregnancy-induced hypertension risk factor, 465
  as preterm birth risk factor, 368, 461
  as spontaneous abortion risk factor, 368, 450

Small-for-gestational age infants, 462–463, 464
Smelting, paternal exposure during, 367
Soldering, maternal exposure during, 460
Solvents, 373
  maternal exposure to
    as cardiovascular malformation risk factor, 479, 480–481
    as congenital abnormalities risk factor, 477, 479, 480–481
    as dysmenorrhea risk factor, 368, 438
    as low birthweight risk factor, 464
    as pregnancy-induced hypertension risk factor, 465
    as preterm birth risk factor, 462
    as spontaneous abortion risk factor, 368, 447–450, 451, 459–460
  parental exposure to, as childhood cancer risk factor, 499–514
  paternal exposure to, 367, 368, 487, 489, 490
  as pesticide components, 473
Sperm, chemical and physical agent exposures of, 515
Spermatoxins, 365
Sperm counts, decrease of, 364, 365
Sperm motility
  analysis of, 391–392, 394
  heavy metals-related impairment of, 367
Standardized fertility ratio, 436
  birth rate overestimation by, 408
Steroids, spermatogenesis-impairing effect of, 389
Stress
  as menstrual disorder risk factor, 438
  as preterm birth risk factor, 461
Subfertility, occupational exposure-related, 440–441
  methodologic issues in, 436–437
Surveillance programs
  of paternal occupational exposure, 411
  of workplace reproductive hazards, 544, 545

Teratology studies, developmental neurotoxicity guidelines for, 375–376
Testes
  biopsy of, 399
  physical examination of, 390
Testosterone, in male infertility, 399
Tetrachloroethylene, maternal exposure to, as spontaneous abortion risk factor, 449
Textiles, parental exposure to, as childhood cancer risk factor, 515, 526–528
Threshold limit values (TLVs), 374, 379
Thyroid disease, as infertility risk factor, 389
Time to conception, 435, 436

Tobacco use, spermatogenesis-impairing effect of, 389
Toluene
  as congenital abnormalities risk factor, 477
  maternal exposure to, as spontaneous abortion risk factor, 447, 449, 450, 459–460
  as menstrual disorder risk factor, 438
Toluene diamine, 406
Tort cases, reproductive hazard-related
  International Union of United Auto Workers v. *Johnson Controls, Inc.*, 379, 381, 546, 547, 548
  litigation outcomes of, 547–548
  proof of causation in, 545
  for workers' compensation claims, 547
Toxic Substances Control Act, 374, 383
Trichloroethylene, as spontaneous abortion risk factor, 459–460
Trichloromethane, as spontaneous abortion risk factor, 449
Trophoblastic hormone metabolites, urinary assays of, 424
Tuberculosis, as infertility risk factor, 389
Turner's syndrome, 418

Unions, male/female membership of, 364
Union workers, spontaneous abortion in, 454
United Auto Workers, fetal protection policy lawsuit by, 379, 381, 546, 547, 548
Urinary tract cancers, parental occupational exposure-related
  agricultural employment-related, 514, 519
  manufacturing chemicals exposure-related, 499, 511–512, 514
  metals exposure-related, 524–525
  textiles exposure-related, 528
  wood-related occupations employment-related, 532–533
Urine assays, for female reproductive health evaluation, **423–433**
  to detect early fetal loss, 368, 425–426
  to monitor ovarian function, 368, 426–431
  to monitor pituitary function, 431

Varicocele, 390, 393
Vasography, 399
VDTs (video display terminals), maternal exposure to, 373, 483–484
  as low birthweight risk factor, 464
  as pregnancy-induced hypertension risk factor, 465
  as preterm birth risk factor, 461–462
  as spontaneous abortion risk factor, 444–446, 459
Venereal disease, as infertility risk factor, 389
Vietnam veterans, 410, 474

Warning labels, for toxic materials, 543
Water beds
    as low birthweight risk factor, 463–464
    as spontaneous abortion risk factor, 446
Welding, paternal exposure during, 367, 368, 487
Wilms' tumor, parental occupational exposure-
        related, 514, 515
Women. *See also* Maternal exposure
    labor force participation by, 364
Wood-related occupations, parental
        employment in, as childhood cancer risk
        factor, 515, 532–533

Workers' compensation, 380, 547
Work force, demographics of, 364–365
Working poor, demographics of, 364–365
Workplace policy, on reproductive health
        hazards, **541–549**
    elements of, 542–545
    legal and ethical issues in, 545–548

Xylene
    as menstrual disorder risk factor,
        438
    paternal exposure to, 490